THE
HOW NOT TO DIE
COOKBOOK

THE
HOW NO
COOKBOOK

MICHAEL GREGER, M.D., FACLM

WITH Gene Stone
RECIPES BY Robin Robertson

T TO DIE

bluebird
books for life

First published in the US 2017 by Flatiron Books

First published as hardback in the UK 2017 by Macmillan

This edition first published 2018 by Bluebird
an imprint of Pan Macmillan
20 New Wharf Road, London N1 9RR
Associated companies throughout the world
www.panmacmillan.com

ISBN 978-1-5290-1081-7

Photography by Antonis Achilleos

Interior design by Alison Lew/Vertigo Design NYC

Cover design by James Annal

Cover photography by Antonis Achilleos

Printed and bound in Italy

Visit **www.panmacmillan.com** to read more about all our books
and to buy them. You will also find features, author interviews and
news of any author events, and you can sign up for e-newsletters
so that you're always first to hear about our new releases.

CONTENTS

Introduction viii

The Daily Dozen xx

ONE **SIMPLE PREPARATIONS** 1

TWO **BREAKFAST** 10

THREE **SNACKS, DIPS AND SPREADS** 28

FOUR **SOUPS AND CHILLIES** 46

FIVE **SALADS AND DRESSINGS** 68

SIX **BURGERS, WRAPS AND MORE** 86

SEVEN **VERY VEGGIE MAINS** 102

EIGHT **BEAN CUISINE** 122

NINE **GREAT GRAINS** 140

TEN **SIDES** 162

ELEVEN **SWEETS** 184

TWELVE **SIPS** 204

Sample Menus for 14 Days 220

Kitchen Techniques 225

Shopping and Stocking the Cupboards 227

References 230

Index 237

INTRODUCTION

I admit it.

I am a nutrition nerd. I love digging through the scientific literature for the fun of it, for the sheer fascination of how our body works, for all the puzzles to be solved. In high school, I used to skip class to hang out in the science library at the local university, spending countless hours trying to read the new issues of all the journals. I hardly understood any of it, but I just loved the whole concept of scientific inquiry: using experimental evidence to test our theories about the universe.

In college, I pursued a biophysics major. I was most interested in the mysteries of the universe inside each of us. As enthralling as all of science and mathematics was, I came to realize that our number one cause of death and disability wasn't the Higgs boson − it was our diet. My mother's deep involvement in the civil rights movement inspired me to dedicate my life to making the world a better place, and my grandmother's miraculous recovery from end-stage heart disease, due to a change in her diet, provided the direction: I would become a doctor and specialize in nutrition.

Even if it didn't help a soul, though, I could happily spend seven days a week lost in the dusty stacks of some medical library basement to satisfy my own curiosity. But what most motivates me every morning to jump out of bed (and onto my treadmill desk!) are all the lives I'm able to help change and save with the information I uncover. For years, my work had touched millions through NutritionFacts.org, but it wasn't until *How Not to Die* was published that the deluge started. My inbox, mailbox and voicemail box have been flooded with profound expressions of gratitude from readers telling me how the science I've shared has helped them and their families become healthier. They are such a gift.

Even better is to experience that appreciation for my work face-to-face and heart-to-heart. As I've traveled around the world to share the book, I've been witness to countless stories of transformation. So many people line up to talk with me after my lectures that sometimes it can be several hours before I can dash back to the airport.

The stories often shared with me are not the ones most doctors hear, tales of pain and sickness. These are stories of regained health and happy endings. What could be more satisfying − for both of us?

Let me share one of these stories with you.

I met Chris, a middle-aged man, after a presentation I gave in Boston at Harvard's Dana-Farber Cancer Institute, where he was employed. Chris had come to my talk because although his type 2 diabetes diagnosis was about ten years old, he wasn't willing to settle for a lifetime of medication and monitoring as his doctor contended was to be his fate.

His physician had told him his diabetes was probably just the result of bad genes and Chris would need to take pills, adding he should 'watch his sugar' (whatever that means). Chris knew diabetes was linked to such complications as blindness and amputations, and his doctor didn't seem very optimistic about the prognosis, nor did he offer any other recommendations.

Ten years earlier, Chris left his doctor's office feeling hopeless and helpless. He felt that he had just been given a death sentence. But he never stopped trying to seek out other answers, which brought him to my lecture.

After Chris recounted his experience, I told him that despite what his doctor might think, we actually have tremendous power over our health destiny. The vast majority of premature death and disability is preventable with a plant-based diet and other healthy lifestyle changes, and type 2 diabetes is a perfect example of a correctable disease.

Chris then handed me a copy of *How Not to Die* to autograph. As I always do when signing books, I included my personal e-mail address and cell phone number, and encouraged him to contact me if there was anything I could do to help him or his family.

About ten months later, Chris sent me this e-mail:

> Dear Doc,
> You won't believe this. My diabetes is GONE. I beat it, doc! How Not to Die *really did save my life! Guess what else? My wife has had problems with her weight since she was a teenager. We went on a plant-based diet together, and she has, for the first time in years, gotten to a normal weight! We are both so happy, we feel like teenagers again. (Did I tell you we were high school sweethearts? That was a very long time ago, but it doesn't feel so long ago anymore!)*
>
> *Also I want to mention that this diet is saving us some serious cash! I used to spend over $70 per month on my diabetes medications, my sugar meter, and test strip supplies. Now we are putting that money saved on medicine into . . . guess what . . . a Happiness Savings Account!*
>
> *We have both always wanted a dog, and when I finally beat diabetes, my wife said, 'Your getting your health back is the best day of my life. We should celebrate it.' And I told her I wanted to go to the shelter and get a dog. When the staff at the shelter asked what kind of dog we wanted, I said, 'A nice dog who you don't think anyone else will want. The dog who everyone else gave up on. Second-chance dog, that's MY dog, please.'*
>
> *The shelter folks talked for a minute, and then they brought out a big black dog with her head down and her tail tucked between her legs. We took one look at each other. Found out her name was Joy. Strange name for a sad dog, right? Well, we bonded fast, and now Joy, my wife, and I walk together every morning. We call it our JoyWalk! Joy is now living up to her name, and I think she saved me as much as I saved her.*
>
> *Most days I find all these new healthy choices easy, but when I get sidetracked, I just look at my Joy and remember how things were, and I remind myself that we are never going back there.*
>
> *Thank you for talking to me and for caring about me and my family. You will never know how much it means to me. I hope you can tell everyone what you told me about genes NOT being our destiny. There is hope and (at least in my house) there is Joy! Thanks, Dr. Greger!*

You're welcome, Chris!

Not everyone is so magnanimous, though. Others are angry. Why didn't their doctor tell them about how lifesaving our dietary choices can be? When I present decades-old studies showing how easily some of our leading killers can be reversed, the audience is left thinking, 'Wait a second. Does that mean my brother didn't have to die?!' Or their sister or mother or best friend. Dr. Dean Ornish was publishing studies back in the 1990s proving heart disease could be reversed.[1] The diabetes reversal study I presented at the event Chris attended was published in 1979. It showed that people who had been living with type 2 diabetes for as long as twenty years, injecting up to 32 units of insulin a day, could get off all their insulin in as few as thirteen days.[2]

Let that sink in for a moment: People with diabetes for twenty years can go off all insulin in less than two weeks. They endured diabetes for twenty years because no one had told them about a plant-based diet. For decades, they had been just thirteen days away from being free . . . .

• • •

Although it technically is one, I don't think of this as a vegetarian cookbook. Eating healthfully is not about vegetarianism, veganism, or any other '-ism'. From a nutrition standpoint, the reason I don't like the terms *vegetarian* and *vegan* is that they are defined by what you *don't* eat. Too often I meet vegans who proudly tell me about their animal-free diet . . . which seems to be composed primarily of French fries, fake meat and nondairy ice cream. That

menu may be vegan, but it isn't particularly health-promoting.

This is why I prefer the term *whole-food, plant-based nutrition*. The best available balance of evidence suggests the healthiest diet is one that minimizes the intake of meat, eggs, dairy and processed junk, and maximizes the intake of fruits, vegetables, legumes (beans, split peas, chickpeas and lentils), whole grains, nuts and seeds, mushrooms, and herbs and spices – basically, real food that grows out of the ground. Those are our healthiest choices.

What do I mean by *whole food*? I mean a food that is not overly processed. In other words, nothing bad has been added, and nothing good has been taken away.

A classic example of food processing is the milling of grains, such as transforming whole wheat into white flour or 'polishing' brown rice into white rice. White rice may have a clean look, but it's also practically devoid of the essential nutrients found in brown rice, such as B vitamins. Before food manufacturers started refortifying white rice with vitamins, millions of people died from beriberi, a vitamin B-deficiency disease that resulted from eating nutritionally empty white rice. Even though refined grains are now typically fortified with a few vitamins, they are still deficient in all the myriad phytonutrients found in the whole grain.

Using my definition of *nothing bad added, nothing good taken away*, I consider pinhead oats, rolled oats and even (plain) instant oatmeal relatively unprocessed, though the best option whenever possible is whole, intact grains.

By *plant-based*, I mean centering one's diet on as many whole plant foods as possible. For

How Not to Die, I created a traffic-light system to classify the Green Light foods people should eat more of, the Yellow Light foods we should eat less of, and the Red Light foods we should ideally avoid on a daily basis. It matters little what healthy folks eat on their birthday, holidays and special occasions. It's the day-to-day stuff that adds up. As Kaiser Permanente's guide *The Plant-Based Diet: A Healthier Way to Eat* puts it: 'If you find you cannot do a plant-based diet 100 percent of the time, then aim for 80 percent. Any movement toward more plants and fewer animal products [and processed foods] can improve your health!'[3]

I've tried to ensure all the recipes in this book are composed only of Green Light ingredients. This is not to say that all processed foods are bad for you. Foods are not so much good or bad as they are better or worse. Unprocessed foods tend to be more healthful than processed ones. Think of it this way: adding almonds to your oatmeal is better than putting almond milk on it, whereas almond milk would be better than putting dairy milk on it.

• • •

How Not to Die was inspired by my remarkable grandmother who was told at just sixty-five years old that her life was over. Her doctors sent her home in a wheelchair to die. However, soon after being discharged from the hospital, she was watching television and saw a *60 Minutes* segment about Nathan Pritikin, who was a pioneer in reversing heart disease through eating a plant-based diet. My grandmother flew to Pritikin's center in California to see whether his plan might help her. They wheeled her in, and she walked out on her own two feet, healthy. She was able to live thirty-one additional years beyond her death sentence – to continue to enjoy life with her six grandkids, including me.

This book was inspired by you, my readers and supporters, who have asked me so often about my favorite recipes, specific recommendations on meal planning, and the best ways to get as many of the Daily Dozen into your life as possible. I hope I can do for your family what Pritikin did for mine.

THE HOW NOT TO DIE APPROACH

For those of you who have not yet read or listened to *How Not to Die*, I encourage you to pick up a copy at your local bookstore or library. I have no personal financial stake in book sales. All the proceeds I receive from sales of any of my books, DVDs and speaking engagements are donated to charity. So, it's not for personal gain that I hope you'll check out my last book. I truly believe it can help you live a healthier and happier life.

What follows here is a very brief summary of *How Not to Die*'s subject matter. This quick synopsis will help you understand the reason I've included these specific (and delicious) recipes in this companion cookbook – they all contain the whole plant foods that may be most helpful in warding off disease and restoring health.

• • •

In the late 1950s, forty-one-year-old engineer Nathan Pritikin was diagnosed with coronary heart disease. His doctors told him there was nothing he could do but take lots of naps, avoid stairs and spend as much time as possible with his family. But instead of waiting for the inevitable, Pritikin took matters into his own hands and devoured everything he could find on his disease. His research eventually inspired him to adopt a plant-based diet, and within two years, his cholesterol plummeted from over 300 to below 160. Rather than dropping dead from a heart attack, Pritikin went on to help countless others reverse their own heart disease. One was my grandma who, as detailed in Pritikin's biography, became one of his most famous success stories.[4]

My grandmother's miraculous recovery is what inspired me to go to medical school. When I got there, however, I was shocked to find out this whole body of evidence on reversing chronic disease with lifestyle changes – opening up arteries without drugs or surgery – was largely being ignored by mainstream medicine. If effectively the *cure* to our leading cause of death could get lost down the rabbit hole and ignored, what other information might be buried in the medical literature? I made it my life's mission to find out. That's what led me to start NutritionFacts.org and that's what led me to write *How Not to Die*.

Plant-based nutrition is the only diet that's ever been proven to reverse heart disease in the majority of patients. If that's all a plant-based diet could do – reverse our number one killer – then shouldn't that be the default diet until proven otherwise? Even more so, since it can also be effective in treating, arresting, and reversing some of our other leading killers as well.

In *How Not to Die*, I cover the role diet may play in preventing and reversing each of the fifteen leading causes of premature death. Here they are, in order, starting with the most common condition, and the one my grandma was able to reverse so successfully.

CORONARY HEART DISEASE. Our number one killer lays waste to 375,000 Americans each year.[5] But, as the China-Cornell-Oxford Project suggested, it doesn't have to be that way. Led by Professor Emeritus T. Colin Campbell, this exhaustive study examined the dietary habits and mortality rates of several hundred thousand rural Chinese and later became the basis for Dr. Campbell's best-selling book *The China Study*. Amazingly, Campbell and colleagues found that many of our Western epidemics of chronic disease, including coronary heart disease, were absent among plant-based Chinese populations.[6] Similar studies conducted early in the twentieth century in rural Africa found the same thing: plant-based populations appeared to suffer one hundred times fewer heart attacks compared to Americans of the same age.[7]

Autopsies of accidental death victims have revealed that heart disease begins very early in life.[8] In fact, heart disease may even begin in the womb if your mother had high cholesterol.[9] In 1953, a study in the *Journal of the American Medical Association* examined three hundred fallen American soldiers from the Korean War, with an average age of twenty-two. The researchers found that 77 percent of the soldiers already had visible evidence of coronary atherosclerosis, and some even had arteries that were blocked off by 90 percent or more.[10] Other studies of accidental death victims have shown that fatty streaks – the precursor to plaque buildup – tend to appear by age ten among those eating the standard American diet.[11]

We couldn't be sure it was the food, though, until it was put to the test. Dr. Dean Ornish was the first to prove in a randomized controlled trial that a plant-based diet and other healthy lifestyle changes could reverse heart disease.[12] Dr. Caldwell Esselstyn Jr. followed up using just the dietary component. In 2014, he published a study involving nearly two hundred patients with severe heart disease – some like my grandma who couldn't make it to the mailbox without being crippled over in pain. At the onset of the trial, Dr. Esselstyn told his patients to adopt a whole-food, plant-based diet. After making the switch, more than 99 percent of his compliant patients avoided further major cardiac events.[13]

LUNG DISEASES. Lung cancer, chronic obstructive pulmonary disease (COPD) and asthma collectively kill 296,000 Americans every year.[14] A plant-based diet may be able to help prevent all three. While the best way to prevent lung cancer is to avoid smoking, a single stalk of broccoli per day can boost the activity of detoxifying enzymes in the liver, helping to prevent lung-cancer – causing DNA damage at the cellular level.[15] Each daily serving of fruit is associated with men having a 24 percent lower risk of dying from COPD – a condition including emphysema that makes it difficult to breathe and gets worse over time. Finally, high vegetable consumption is associated with just half the odds of children developing asthma.[17] As far as treating asthma, simply adding a few more servings of fruits and vegetables to your diet has been shown in a randomized controlled trial to cut asthma attacks in half.[18]

BRAIN DISEASES. The two most serious brain diseases are stroke and Alzheimer's, which collectively kill 215,000 Americans each year.[19] Both have touched my life: my mom's father died of a stroke, and her mother of Alzheimer's. With most strokes, blood flow to the brain is cut off, depriving it of oxygen. The consequences wrought by a stroke depend on which area of the brain was damaged. People who experience a brief stroke might only need to contend with arm or leg weakness, whereas those who suffer a major stroke can be struck with paralysis, lose the ability to speak, or, as is too often the case, die.

Fortunately, a plant-based diet may reduce the odds of a stroke. Increasing intake of fiber (which is found only in plants) by only 7 grams per day – that's about a cup of raspberries – is associated with a 7 percent risk reduction.[20] In addition, a meta-analysis in the *Journal of the American College of Cardiology* found that increasing your potassium intake by 1,640 mg – a cup (225g) of cooked greens or a half-cup (35g) of beans – was associated with a 21 percent reduction in stroke risk.[21]

Alzheimer's, a horrendous disease that destroys our memory and sense of self, can neither be cured nor treated effectively. However, there is an emerging consensus that the same foods that clog our arteries can also clog our brain. A senior scientist at the Center for Alzheimer's Research entitled a review article 'Alzheimer's Disease Is Incurable but Preventable'.[22] Autopsies have shown repeatedly that Alzheimer's patients tend to have significantly more atherosclerotic plaque buildup and narrowing of the arteries within the brain.[23]

Numerous studies have shown that Alzheimer's is not a primarily genetic disease. For example, the Alzheimer's rates among Japanese men living in the United States are much higher than those of Japanese men living in Japan.[24] The same goes for African Americans in Indianapolis compared to Africans in Nigeria.[25] The problem may be the typical American diet, which can choke the arteries within the brain. Where is the world's lowest validated rate of Alzheimer's? Rural northern India,[26] where people traditionally eat a plant-based diet centered on grains and vegetables.[27]

DIGESTIVE CANCERS. Every year, 106,000 Americans die from cancers that might well have been prevented.[28] While some cancers have a significant genetic component, common digestive cancers are more likely the result of poor dietary choices. If you were to flatten out your intestines, they could cover thousands of square feet.[29] This means an extraordinary amount of surface area interacts with your food as it travels through your digestive tract. Food is our single greatest exposure to the outside environment. Colorectal (colon and rectal) cancer is one of the most commonly diagnosed cancers in the United States, but it's relatively rare in India. Comparatively, American men have eleven times more colorectal cancer diagnoses and women have ten times more.[30] One possible reason? Spices, such as turmeric, a staple of Indian cuisine, including curry powder, appear to have a variety of anticancer properties.[31] Another possibility is the food in which the turmeric-laden curry powder is used: India is one of the world's largest producers of fruits and vegetables, and only about 7 percent of the adult population eats meat on a daily basis. What most of this population does eat daily are legumes (beans, split peas, chickpeas and lentils) and dark green, leafy vegetables,[32] which are packed with another class of cancer-fighting compounds called phytates.

Pancreatic cancer is among the most lethal cancers, with only 6 percent of patients surviving five years after diagnosis.[33] This is why prevention is paramount. The National Institutes of Health – AARP study, which followed 525,000 people aged fifty to seventy-one for years beginning in 1995, found the consumption of fat from animal sources was significantly associated with pancreatic cancer risk. No such correlation was found with consuming plant fats.[34] Likewise, the European Prospective Investigation into Cancer and Nutrition (EPIC) study, which followed 477,000 people for a decade beginning in 1992, found a 72 percent increased risk of pancreatic cancer for every 50 grams of poultry (about a quarter of a chicken breast) consumed daily.[35]

INFECTIONS. With each breath, we take in thousands of bacteria. With each bite of food comes millions more. Most microbes are harmless, but some cause serious infections, such as influenza and pneumonia, which alone kill fifty-seven thousand Americans each year.[36] A plant-based diet may be able to boost your immunity to keep you safer. In a 2012 study published in the *American Journal of Clinical Nutrition,* elderly volunteers who were randomized to eat five or more servings of fruit and vegetables daily had an 82 percent greater protective antibody response to a pneumonia vaccine compared to those who ate two or fewer servings a day.[37] In other words, you can bolster your immune system function just by eating more produce. Broccoli and other cruciferous vegetables have been shown to boost the effectiveness of intraepithelial lymphocytes, a special type of white blood cell that is the first line of gut defense against pathogens.[38] Blueberries, meanwhile, have been shown to almost double our levels of natural killer cells, which are vital members of the immune system's rapid response team against viruses and cancer cells.[39]

TYPE 2 DIABETES. More than twenty million Americans are currently diagnosed with diabetes, the 'Black Death of the twenty-first century' – a tripling of cases since 1990.[40] Diabetes currently causes about 50,000 cases of kidney failure, 75,000 lower extremity amputations, 650,000 cases of vision loss, and about 75,000 deaths every year in the United States.[41] Type 2 diabetes is caused by our body's resistance to the effects of insulin, a vital hormone that shuttles glucose (blood sugar) into our cells, thereby preventing dangerous levels from accumulating in the blood. This insulin resistance is primarily caused by a fatty buildup inside our muscle cells.[42] This fat can come from excess fat in our diet or from excess fat on our body. Up to 90 percent of people who develop diabetes are overweight.[43]

A plant-based diet can help keep off the pounds. There appears to be a step-wise drop in obesity rates as one moves from nonvegetarian diets to flexitarian (part-time vegetarian) diets to pescatarian (fish-eating vegetarian) to vegetarian to vegan. Those eating strictly plant-based were the only dietary group that was on average at an ideal weight, with an average body mass index (BMI) of 23.6. (A BMI over 25 is considered overweight.) Nonvegetarians topped the charts at an unhealthy 28.8.[44] If you are trying to lose weight, including plant-based foods in your diet could help you: simply adding beans to diets was found to be as effective at slimming waistlines and improving blood sugar markers as calorie-cutting portion control.[45]

Based on a study of tens of thousands of adults in the United States and Canada, people who cut out all animal products, including fish, dairy and eggs, appear to have a 78 percent reduced risk of diabetes.[46] If you already have diabetes, a plant-based diet may even reverse it. Even without weight loss, a plant-based diet can enable those who have had type 2 diabetes for decades get off all their insulin injections in as few as two weeks.[47] That's why if you're on medications to lower blood sugar or blood pressure, it's critical that you make these healthy changes under close medical supervision, so you can be rapidly weaned off these drugs if necessary. Otherwise the diet can work so well that your blood sugars or blood pressure can drop too low. Once your body has a chance to start healing itself, you can find yourself overmedicated very quickly.

HIGH BLOOD PRESSURE. Also known as hypertension, high blood pressure is the number one risk factor for death and disability worldwide,[48] laying waste to nine million people each year globally[49] and sixty-five thousand in the United States.[50] Increased blood pressure puts strain on your heart, can damage the sensitive blood vessels in your eyes and kidneys, and cause bleeding in the brain. Many doctors are under the impression that increased blood pressure is a natural consequence of aging, just like getting gray hair and wrinkles – after all, 65 percent of Americans over age sixty can expect to be diagnosed with hypertension.[51] But we've known for nearly a century that blood pressure can remain stable throughout life or actually decrease after age sixty.[52]

On average, high blood pressure medications reduce the risk of heart attack by 15 percent and the risk of stroke by about 25 percent.[53] But in a randomized, controlled trial, three portions of whole grains a day were able

to help people achieve this same benefit without medication.[54] A cup of hibiscus herbal tea with each meal can lower systolic blood pressure by 6 points compared to a control group.[55] A double-blind, placebo-controlled, randomized trial found people with hypertension who consumed a few spoonfuls of flaxseeds every day for six months lowered their blood pressure on average from 158/82 to 143/75. That could be expected to result in 46 percent fewer strokes and 29 percent less heart disease over time.[56]

LIVER DISEASE. Many people assume that liver disease, which kills sixty thousand Americans each year,[57] is the result of heavy alcohol consumption or intravenous drug use. But non-alcoholic fatty liver disease (NAFLD) has quietly become the most common cause of chronic liver disease in the United States, afflicting an estimated seventy million people[58] and nearly 100 percent of those who are severely obese.[59] As with alcoholic fatty liver, NAFLD begins with the buildup of fat on the liver. In rare cases, this can cause inflammation and lead to fatal scarring of the liver, called cirrhosis.[60] Drinking just one can of soda per day appears to raise the odds of fatty liver disease by 45 percent.[61] People who eat the meat equivalent of fourteen chicken nuggets daily have nearly triple the rate of NAFLD compared to people who eat seven nuggets' worth or less.[62] One plant-based way to fight liver inflammation: Eating oatmeal was found in a double-blind, randomized, placebo-controlled trial to be able to significantly improve liver function among overweight men and women – and help them lose weight as well.[63]

BLOOD CANCERS. Leukemia, lymphoma and multiple myeloma are sometimes referred to as liquid tumors because the cancer cells often circulate throughout the body rather than get concentrated in a solid mass. Every year these cancers kill fifty-six thousand Americans.[64] One of the largest studies on diet and cancer found that people who consume a more plant-based diet are less likely to develop all forms of cancer combined, with the greatest apparent protection against blood cancers.[65] The Iowa Women's Health Study, which has followed more than thirty-five thousand women for decades, showed that higher broccoli or other cruciferous vegetable intake was associated with a lower risk of non-Hodgkin's lymphoma.[66] This is consistent with a study at the Mayo Clinic that found people who ate about three or more servings of green, leafy vegetables per week appeared to have only about half the odds of getting lymphoma compared with those who ate less than one serving a week.[67] This protection may be due to the high antioxidant content of plant foods. It's important to note that this benefit is not found for antioxidant supplements.

KIDNEY DISEASE. Your kidneys filter 150 quarts of blood every twenty-four hours to produce the 1 to 2 quarts of urine you pee out each day. If the kidneys aren't functioning correctly, metabolic waste products can accumulate in the blood and eventually lead to dangerous problems, including weakness, shortness of breath, confusion, and abnormal heart rhythms. Eventually they can fail altogether, resulting in death unless regular dialysis is performed — a fate that befalls nearly forty-seven thousand Americans each year.[68]

A recent national survey found that only 41 percent of Americans tested had normal kidney function.[69] Most people with kidney disease may not even know they are suffering from it.[70] Researchers at Harvard University followed the diet and kidney function of thousands of healthy women for more than a decade. They concluded that three specific dietary components are associated with declining kidney function: animal protein, animal fat, and cholesterol.[71] Each is found only in one place: animal products.

Animal protein triggers an inflammatory reaction in the kidneys.[72] Within hours of your consuming meat, your kidneys rev up into hyperfiltration mode.[73] (*Hyperfiltration* means that your kidneys start to work overtime as increasing pressure builds up within them.) A lifetime of overeating animal protein may take its toll on your kidneys, causing them to be less and less efficient as you age. But your kidneys can handle the same amount of plant protein without a problem.[74] Plant protein may even help preserve function in ailing kidneys.[75]

BREAST CANCER. Killing forty thousand American women each year,[76] breast cancer is among the most feared diagnoses a woman can receive — and what we eat matters. The Long Island Breast Cancer Study Project found that postmenopausal women eating more grilled, barbecued, or smoked meats over their lifetime were associated with as much as 47 percent higher odds of breast cancer.[77] In the largest study on cholesterol and cancer to date — with more than a million participants — a 17 percent increased breast cancer risk was found in premenopausal women who had total cholesterol levels over 240 compared with women whose cholesterol was under 160.[78] This means that the same plant-based diet that helps lower a woman's risk of heart disease may also help lower her risk of breast cancer. The Black Women's Health Study, which followed fifty thousand African American women beginning in 1995, found that women who ate two or more servings of vegetables a day had a significantly decreased risk of a kind of breast cancer that's hard to treat: estrogen-receptor-negative and progesterone-receptor-negative.[79] In premenopausal women, a high-fiber diet was associated with an extraordinary 85 percent lower odds of that type of estrogen-receptor-negative breast tumors.[80]

SUICIDAL DEPRESSION. Forty-one thousand Americans take their life every year,[81] and depression is a leading cause.[82] While anyone experiencing suicidal thoughts should seek professional help, lifestyle interventions can help heal the mind as well as the body. One way to fight the blues may be with greens: higher consumption of vegetables may cut the odds of developing depression by as much as 62 percent.[83] In general, eating lots of fruits and veggies may present 'a non-invasive, natural, and inexpensive therapeutic means to support a healthy brain'.[84] Additionally, the spice saffron was found to be as effective at treating mild to moderate depression as the antidepressant drug Prozac[85] – and it tastes a lot better.

PROSTATE CANCER. Prostate cancer is much more common than most people think: autopsy studies have shown that about half of men over the age of eighty suffer from it.[86] Most die of other diseases first, but prostate cancer still

kills twenty-eight thousand men every year.[87] Recent studies have revealed a link between diet and prostate cancer. Population studies have suggested the prevalence of prostate cancer increases as animal consumption increases. For example, the death rate of prostate cancer in Japan has increased twenty-five-fold since World War II, and this dramatic spike coincides with a twenty-fold increase in dairy consumption, a seven-fold increase in egg consumption and a nine-fold increase in meat consumption.[88] Dairy consumption has been consistently associated with risk: a 2015 meta-analysis and review found that high intakes of dairy products – milk and cheese (including low- and non-fat varieties) but not nondairy sources of calcium – appear to increase total prostate cancer risk.[89]

If you have early-stage prostate cancer, you may be able to reverse its progression with a plant-based diet. After conquering our number-one killer, heart disease, Dr. Dean Ornish moved on to killer number two, cancer. Prostate cancer patients were randomized into two groups: a control group that wasn't given any diet or lifestyle advice beyond whatever their personal doctors told them to do, and a healthy-living group prescribed a plant-based diet centered on fruits, vegetables, whole grains and beans, along with other healthy lifestyle behaviors. After a year, the control group's blood PSA – a marker of prostate cancer growth inside the body – tended to increase, but the plant-based group's PSA levels tended to go down,[90] which suggests their prostate tumors actually shrank. No surgery, no chemotherapy, no radiation – just eating and living healthily.

PARKINSON'S DISEASE. A disease of prizefighters and NFL linebackers who sustain repeated head trauma, Parkinson's disease, which kills twenty-five thousand Americans every year,[91] may also be due to brain damage caused by exposure to pollutants and toxic heavy metals that build up in the food supply. Poultry and tuna have been found to be the leading food sources of arsenic; dairy, the number one source of lead; and seafood, including tuna, the number one source of mercury.[92] An analysis of more than twelve thousand food and feed samples across twenty countries found that the highest contamination of the toxic chemical polychlorinated biphenyl (PCB) was found in fish and fish oil, followed by eggs, dairy and then other meats. The lowest contamination was found at the bottom of the food chain, in plants.[93] Those who eat a plant-based diet have been found to have significantly lower blood levels of a PCB implicated in increasing the risk of developing Parkinson's disease.[94]

Wait a minute, Doc, some of you eagle-eyed readers might be thinking. *That's only fourteen.* Indeed! The fifteenth killer is actually the third-leading cause of death, responsible for 225,000 deaths annually.[95] Oh, and it's not a disease.

It's doctors.

That's right. Medical care is the third-leading cause of death. Whether it's death caused by a hospital infection,[96] unnecessary surgery, receiving the wrong medication, or an adverse side effect from the right medication,[97] the sad reality is that you can head into a routine procedure and never return home. While hospitals are striving to reduce medical error and the spread of infections, they remain dangerous places.[98] Did you know that getting a routine chest CT scan is estimated to inflict the same cancer risk as smoking seven hundred cigarettes?[99] Or that 1 middle-aged woman in every 270 may develop cancer after a single CT angiogram?[100] Or that when it comes to cholesterol, blood pressure, and blood-thinning drugs, the chance of even high-risk patients benefiting from them is typically less than 5 percent over a period of five years?[101] Doctors and patients alike wildly overestimate the power of pills and procedures to ward off death and disability.

To me, the true tragedy is all the lost opportunities to address the root causes of chronic disease. Our modern medical system is great at fixing broken bones and curing infections, but it fails woefully at preventing and reversing the most common causes of death. Until the system changes, we have to take personal responsibility for our own health and our family's. We can't wait until society catches up to the science, because it's a matter of life and death. I wrote *How Not to Die* to help you understand the role foods can play in preventing, arresting, or reversing the fifteen leading causes of death. I wrote this book to help you actually do it, right in your own kitchen.

THE DAILY DOZEN

Many have told me *How Not to Die* is their nutrition 'bible'.

I've been honored to hear from countless lay-people who've shared their enthusiasm for *How Not to Die*, and high school students to graduate students – even professors – have told me they've used it as their go-to source for papers and lectures. Yes, I cite thousands of peer-reviewed papers from the scientific literature, but I didn't want to just write a reference book. I also wanted to create a practical guide on translating this mountain of evidence into easy-to-make, day-to-day decisions, and that's how I shaped the second half of the book. I center my recommendations around a Daily Dozen check-list of all the things I try to fit into my daily routine and encourage you to, as well.

And, yes: There's an app for that. 'Dr. Greger's Daily Dozen' is available as a free app for Android and iPhone. The app specifies serving sizes and can help you keep track of how you're doing.

For my family, the Daily Dozen checklist has been a useful reminder to try to make each meal as healthful as possible. I was so heartened to find out that others found it helpful, too. I've gotten literally thousands of emails from people who excitedly tell me how many check marks they're up to that day.

'I eat more cruciferous vegetables than I ever thought possible,' one woman told me, 'and I never even knew the word *cruciferous* before!' Other people say that ground flaxseeds are now such a basic part of their life that they pack a containerful when they travel. Others tell me they'd never cooked with spices until they read the book, but now that they do, they not only reap the health benefits of turmeric, oregano and the rest, but also find that their meals taste better than ever.

Lots of people have made it into a game. To get in all the servings I recommend, you have to tick off 24 checkboxes a day. People kept asking for meal plans and recipes to help them nail the Daily Dozen every day. I love hearing about all the creative ways readers have told me they are trying to incorporate things like beans and greens into breakfast, but many were left wondering how to shop for, prepare and serve them. What they wanted, they said, was a cookbook.

So, here it is: *The How Not to Die Cookbook*. Its purpose is to give you recipes for meals that are delicious, nutritious, and, of course, help you include all of the Daily Dozen in your life as often as possible.

Centering your diet on the Daily Dozen should make it easier to stay healthy. Remember, eating is a zero-sum game. When you decide to eat one food, it means you are choosing not to eat another food. After all, there's only so much you can consume in one day. So, whatever you choose has an opportunity cost.

That means every time you put something in your mouth, it's a lost opportunity to invest in something healthier. Think of it this way: If you had £2,000 in the bank to spend on food, how would you want to use it? Would you lavish it on wonderful meals that let you check off most of the items on the Daily Dozen list? Or would you waste it on buckets of fried chicken and bags of crisps? I'd like to think that if you've picked up this book, you'd choose the former. In reality, you only have about 2,000 calories to 'spend' each day, and each food choice determines whether you are spending them on something that enriches your health, or bankrupts it.

The recipes in this book will give you the opportunity to prepare meals that provide you with the most nutritional bang for your caloric buck. From Mango-Avocado-Kale Salad with Ginger-Sesame Orange Dressing to Black Bean Soup with Quinoa & Kale to Stuffed Portobellos with Herbed Mushroom Gravy, you will find recipes that make your mouth water and keep your body healthy.

NOTE: *The Daily Dozen represents the twelve things I try to make part of my day, every day. This means anything from five servings of a healthy beverage to at least one serving each of berries, flaxseeds, nuts and seeds, and herbs and spices. You will see a list at the end of each recipe telling you which of the Daily Dozen each recipe includes.*

Dr. Greger's Daily Dozen

√√√ **BEANS**

√ **BERRIES**

√√√ **OTHER FRUITS**

√ **CRUCIFEROUS VEGETABLES**

√√ **GREENS**

√√ **OTHER VEGETABLES**

√ **FLAXSEEDS (OR LINSEEDS)**

√ **NUTS AND SEEDS**

√ **HERBS AND SPICES**

√√√ **WHOLE GRAINS**

√√√√√ **BEVERAGES**

√ **EXERCISE**

Here is the Daily Dozen and the number of servings I recommend for each one. For years, I had this list on a little dry-erase board on our refrigerator. Feel free to cut this one out (or make your own copy) and do the same. It's also useful to take with you when you go shopping to guide you through your healthiest choices. And remember, it's just about doing your best. There are times, especially when I am traveling, that I only hit a quarter of my goals. When that happens, I just try to make up for it the next day. The same goes for you: if one day you only get a few of these foods into your diet, the next day, do your best to get more!

SIMPLE PREPARATIONS

Before we dive into the incredible recipes we've created for you, I wanted to first share ten flavor-makers that you'll use in many of the recipes throughout the book. I love them all, but two of my favorites are Savory Spice Blend, a seasoning mix that not only adds enormous zest, but is salt-free, and Umami Sauce, another flavor enhancer that is a delicious alternative to soy sauce preparations such as stir-fries and sautés. Also in this chapter are recipes for making your own almond milk and vegetable broth, a healthy version of Parmesan cheese to sprinkle on pasta dishes, date syrup, balsamic glaze and ranch dressing, as well as simple instructions on how to roast garlic.

ALMOND MILK

DATE SYRUP

SAVORY SPICE BLEND

NUTTY PARM

UMAMI SAUCE

ROASTED GARLIC

VEGETABLE BROTH

RANCH DRESSING

BALSAMIC-DATE GLAZE

HEALTHY HOT SAUCE

HARISSA

- If using dried beans, cook them in large batches and then portion and freeze them. I used to use tinned beans until I discovered how easy it is to prepare dried beans from scratch, using an electric pressure cooker.

- Instead of making one or two servings at a time, cook a large pot of a staple grain or a grain with a quick-cooking legume, such as lentils, mixed in. Then, simply portion and freeze until you want to thaw, heat and enjoy.

- Prepare double batches of recipes for long-cooking dishes, such as stews, soups or chillies. You'll not only save time – you'll get more enhanced flavor when you reheat. They're even better when served later in the week or after being frozen for a time.

- Make seasoning blends, sauces or dressings ahead of time to have on hand.

- Double up on prep, such as chopping onions, when making more than one recipe, so you have enough for both. When you only need half an onion, chop the whole onion and refrigerate the unused portion in a sealed container.

TRAFFIC LIGHT SYSTEM

In *How Not to Die*, I explain what I call Dining by Traffic Light. This is a system that is as easy to follow as obeying a traffic light. Green is for go. Green Light foods, which are unprocessed plant foods, should make up the bulk of our diet. Yellow is for caution. Yellow Light foods include processed plant foods and unprocessed animal foods. Red is for stop, as in stop and think before you put it in your mouth. Red Light foods are the ultraprocessed plant foods and processed animal foods. The more green lights you hit, the faster you'll get to your health destination!

ALMOND MILK

MAKES: ABOUT *2* CUPS/500ML
· DIFFICULTY: *easy*

Here's a fast and easy way to make a whole-food almond milk. For taste and convenience I personally prefer unsweetened soya milk. (I like the flavor of Whole Foods Market's store brand the best.) But I wanted to embrace the challenge of creating recipes containing only Green Light ingredients. This doesn't offer the calcium, vitamin D and B12 fortification of commercial almond milks, but it avoids the added salt and thickeners of questionable safety, such as carrageenan. Choose almond butter made from raw rather than roasted or toasted almonds to decrease exposure to advanced glycation end products. (See page 108.)

2 tablespoons smooth raw almond butter

2 cups/500ml water

Combine the almond butter and water in a high-speed blender and blend until smooth. Transfer the milk to a glass bottle or jar with a tight-fitting lid and chill until ready to serve. Shake well before using.

DATE SYRUP

MAKES: ABOUT *1½* CUPS/370ML
· DIFFICULTY: *easy*

Green Light sweeteners are a little hard to come by. Date sugar, which is simply dried, pulverized dates, can be used as a whole-food, granulated sugar, and blackstrap molasses is a good choice for a healthy liquid sweetener, but it has a strong, sometimes overpowering flavor. We've come up with our own DIY date syrup we hope you'll love as much as we do.

1 cup/175g pitted dates

1 cup/250ml boiling water

1 teaspoon blended peeled lemon (**see sidebar**)

Combine the dates and hot water in a heatproof bowl and set aside for 1 hour to soften the dates. Transfer the dates and water to a high-speed blender. Add the lemon and blend until smooth. Transfer to a glass jar or other airtight container with a tight-fitting lid. Store the syrup in the refrigerator for up to 2 to 3 weeks.

USING BLENDED WHOLE LEMONS AND LIMES

Instead of cooking with lemon or lime juice, use the blended whole fruit to get more nutritional benefit. When you use just the juice, you lose out on the fiber and all the nutrition that was attached to it.

Here's a great time-saver when cooking with blended lemon or lime. Peel and blend a whole lemon and then freeze it in 1-teaspoon portions – a small silicone ice cube tray is ideal for this. Then, grab a cube from the freezer whenever you need it!

SAVORY SPICE BLEND

MAKES: ABOUT ½ CUP/125G · DIFFICULTY: *easy*

I always have this seasoning blend on hand to add flavor to dishes in place of salt.

2 tablespoons nutritional yeast* (or yeast flakes)

1 tablespoon onion powder

1 tablespoon dried parsley

1 tablespoon dried basil

2 teaspoons dried thyme

2 teaspoons garlic powder

2 teaspoons mustard powder

2 teaspoons paprika

½ teaspoon ground turmeric

½ teaspoon celery seeds

Combine all the ingredients in a spice grinder or blender to mix well and pulverize the dried herbs and spices. Transfer the blend to a shaker bottle or jar with a tight-fitting lid. Store in a cool, dry place.

* *I recommend those with Crohn's disease or hidradenitis suppurativa avoid nutritional yeast.*

NUTTY PARM

MAKES: ABOUT 1½ CUPS/150G · DIFFICULTY: *easy*

For a cheesy flavor, sprinkle this on pasta, grain dishes, salads and snacks like popcorn or kale chips.

½ cup/135g almonds

½ cup/135g Brazil nuts

½ cup/75g nutritional yeast* (or yeast flakes)

2 teaspoons Savory Spice Blend (see left)

Combine all the ingredients in a food processor and process until the nuts are finely ground. Transfer to a covered container or shaker and keep refrigerated.

VARIATION: Substitute different nuts for the almonds or Brazil nuts.

UMAMI SAUCE

MAKES: ABOUT *1¼* CUPS/280G · DIFFICULTY: *easy*

Use this sauce in sautés or stir-fries to boost flavor without adding all the sodium of soy sauce. Umami is one of the five basic tastes, even though many people are only learning about it now. This word was created by a Japanese chemist named Kikunae Ikeda from *umai*, which means 'delicious', and *mi*, which means 'taste'. The perfect name, as it is a delicious taste!

1 cup/250ml Vegetable Broth (page 6)

1 teaspoon minced garlic

1 teaspoon grated fresh ginger

1 tablespoon blackstrap molasses

1½ teaspoons Date Syrup (page 3) or date sugar

½ teaspoon jarred tomato purée

½ teaspoon ground black pepper

1½ teaspoons white miso paste blended with 2 tablespoons water

2 teaspoons blended peeled lemon (see page 3)

1 tablespoon rice vinegar*

Heat the broth in a small saucepan over medium heat. Add the garlic and ginger and simmer for 3 minutes. Stir in the molasses, Date Syrup, tomato purée and black pepper and bring just to a boil. Reduce the heat to low and simmer for 1 minute. Remove from the heat, and then stir in the miso mixture, blended lemon and rice vinegar. Taste and adjust the seasonings, if needed. Allow the sauce to cool before transferring to a jar or bottle with a tight-fitting lid or pouring the sauce into an ice cube tray and freezing into individual portions.

* *Vinegar is an honorary Green Light condiment because of the health-promoting benefits of its acetic acid.*

ROASTED GARLIC

MAKES: ABOUT *3* TABLESPOONS
(PER HEAD OF GARLIC) · DIFFICULTY: *easy*

Easy to prepare, roasted garlic adds incredible bursts of flavor to recipes and makes a great spread on toast or sandwiches.

---

1 whole head garlic, or more

Preheat the oven to 400°F/200°C/gas mark 6. Use a sharp knife to cut about ⅓ inch/8mm off the top of a whole garlic head to expose the tops of the garlic cloves. Wrap the garlic head in baking parchment or place in a small covered baking dish, cut side up, and place in the oven. If roasting more than one head of garlic, arrange them, cut side up, in a covered baking dish, or place each head in a separate well of a muffin pan and cover with an inverted baking sheet. Bake for 35 to 45 minutes, or until the garlic cloves are soft and golden brown. Remove from the oven and uncover to let the garlic cool. When the garlic is cool to the touch, gently squeeze each clove individually over a small bowl, allowing the soft, roasted garlic to slip out of the papery skin. (If it is not very soft and golden brown, it needs to be covered or rewrapped in the parchment and baked a few minutes longer.) Enjoy the roasted garlic immediately or store it in the refrigerator in a jar or other container with a tight-fitting lid.

VEGETABLE BROTH

MAKES: ABOUT *6* CUPS/1.4 LITERS
· DIFFICULTY: *easy*

Use this in any of the recipes calling for salt-free vegetable broth.

---

1 medium onion, coarsely chopped

1 carrot, cut into 1-inch/2.5cm pieces

2 celery stalks, coarsely chopped

3 garlic cloves, crushed

2 dried mushrooms

⅓ cup/10g coarsely chopped fresh parsley

½ teaspoon ground black pepper

2 tablespoons white miso paste

Savory Spice Blend (page 4)

In a large pan, heat 1 cup/250ml of water over medium heat. Add the onion, carrot, celery and garlic and cook for 5 minutes. Stir in the mushrooms, parsley and black pepper. Add 7 cups/1.6 liters of water and bring to a boil. Reduce the heat to low and simmer for 1½ hours. Let cool slightly and then transfer to a high-speed blender and blend until smooth. Return the blended broth back to the pan. Ladle about ⅓ cup/80ml of the broth into a small bowl or cup. Add the miso paste and stir well before incorporating into the broth. Add the Savory Spice Blend to taste. Let the broth cool to room temperature; then divide among containers with tight-sealing lids and store in the refrigerator or freezer. Properly stored, the broth will keep for up to 5 days in the refrigerator or up to 3 months in the freezer.

NOTE: If you don't have time to make your own broth, you can buy salt-free vegetable broth or salt-free vegetable bouillon cubes, available in natural food stores or online.

RANCH DRESSING

MAKES: ABOUT *1½* CUPS/340G
· DIFFICULTY: *easy*

Creamy and flavorful, this dressing isn't just for salads. Serve it as a dipping sauce for the Buffalo Cauliflower (page 183), crudités, or anything else you want to kick up a notch.

½ cup/75g raw cashews, soaked for 3 hours and drained

2 cloves Roasted Garlic (page 6)

½ cup/120ml Almond Milk (page 2)

2 tablespoons rice vinegar

2 teaspoons blended peeled lemon (see page 3)

1 tablespoon chopped red onion

2 teaspoons Savory Spice Blend (page 4)

1 teaspoon white miso paste

¾ teaspoon date sugar

1 tablespoon minced fresh parsley

1 teaspoon chopped fresh dill, or ½ teaspoon dried

In a high-speed blender, combine all the ingredients except the parsley and dill, and blend until smooth. Transfer the dressing to a bowl and stir in the parsley and dill. Taste and adjust the seasonings, if needed. (The flavor will get stronger as the dressing sits.) Cover and refrigerate for at least an hour to allow the flavors to develop. Stir or shake before serving.

BALSAMIC-DATE GLAZE

MAKES: ABOUT *1* CUP/250ML · DIFFICULTY: *easy*

Drizzle this rich sauce over Stuffed Sweet Potatoes (page 176), your favorite roasted vegetables or grain dishes, salads and fruits, such as watermelon or strawberries.

½ cup/85g pitted dates
¾ cup/175ml warm water
½ cup/120ml balsamic vinegar

Soften the dates by soaking in warm water for about 10 minutes. In a blender, combine the dates and their soaking water with the balsamic vinegar. Blend until smooth.

Transfer the mixture to a small saucepan and bring to a boil; then reduce the heat to low. Simmer on low until the glaze is reduced and thickened, stirring frequently.

DATES

Growing up, I never liked dates. I thought they were dry and kind of waxy. But then I discovered there were soft, plump, moist varieties that didn't taste like the chalky ones I remembered. Bahri dates – my favorite – are wet and sticky, and when frozen, acquire the taste and chew of caramel candy. Dates are healthy, too: a 2009 study found that eating four to five dried dates per day may improve the antioxidant power of your bloodstream while bringing down triglyceride levels.[103]

HEALTHY HOT SAUCE

MAKES: ABOUT *2* CUPS/450G · DIFFICULTY: *easy*

Most bottled hot sauces contain too much sodium. The good news is, it's easy to make your own – and you can leave out the salt!

12 ounces/350g fresh hot chillies (a single type or mixed), stemmed, halved lengthwise, seeded and chopped
½ cup/75g chopped onion
1 tablespoon minced garlic
½ to 1 cup/120–250ml apple cider vinegar

In a saucepan, combine the chillies, onion, garlic and ¼ cup/60ml of water over high heat. Cook, stirring, for 2 to 3 minutes. Lower the heat to medium-high, add 1¾ cups/425ml of water and continue to cook, stirring occasionally, for 15 to 20 minutes, or until the chillies are very soft. Remove from the heat and let the mixture come to room temperature.

Transfer the chilli mixture to a food processor and process until very smooth. Add ½ cup/120ml of the vinegar and process to blend. Taste the sauce and add more of the vinegar, if desired, to taste. Transfer the hot sauce to a clean glass jar or bottle and secure with an airtight lid. Keep refrigerated. Can be stored in the refrigerator for up to 6 months.

NOTE: Be sure to use rubber gloves when handling hot chillies and do not touch your eyes.

HARISSA

MAKES: ABOUT *1½* CUPS/335G · DIFFICULTY: *easy*

Harissa is an aromatic, spicy paste frequently used in North African and Middle Eastern cooking. It's usually made of hot chilli peppers, garlic, olive oil, and such spices as caraway, coriander, cumin and saffron – but these vary according to preference. Harissa is called the national condiment of Tunisia, where it seems most meals contain it. In the UK, you can find less-than-healthy versions at many supermarkets in tins or jars, which is why I've included a recipe here for you to enjoy.

⅓ cup/10g dried hot red chillies, seeded and cut into small pieces, or to taste

1 tablespoon coriander seeds

2 teaspoons caraway seeds

1 teaspoon cumin seeds

2 roasted red peppers (see above, or shop-bought)

3 garlic cloves, chopped

1 tablespoon nutritional yeast (or yeast flakes)

2 teaspoons white miso paste

Savory Spice Blend (page 4)

Place the dried chillies in a heatproof bowl and cover with boiling water. Set aside for 30 minutes; then drain.

In a small frying pan, stir the coriander, caraway and cumin seeds over low heat until fragrant, about 30 seconds. Transfer to a food processor and add the drained chillies, roasted red peppers, garlic, nutritional yeast, miso and Savory Spice Blend to taste. Process until smooth. Add up to ¼ cup/60ml of water, as needed, to make a smooth, thick sauce.

ROASTING RED PEPPERS

Roast peppers by holding them directly over a gas flame with a pair of tongs until the skin blackens on all sides. They can also be roasted under a grill, turning until the skin blackens all over. Place the blackened peppers in a bowl and cover tightly. Set aside for 10 minutes, or until cool enough to touch with your hands; then remove the blackened skin and the seeds and proceed with the recipe. If you'd rather not roast your own peppers, you can purchase jars of roasted red peppers in supermarkets.

TWO

BREAKFAST

This chapter offers many ways to start your day on the right foot –
even on those days when you get up on the wrong side of the bed.
I like to make whole grains part of my morning routine, whether it's with
oatmeal (with berries or chocolate) or Morning Grain Bowls. When I sit
down with my family, some of our favorite breakfast go-tos are
French Toast with Berry Drizzle, Burrito Breakfast Bake and
Frying Pan Sweet Potato Hash. (If you're looking for smoothies,
you'll find them in the Sips chapter starting on page 204.)

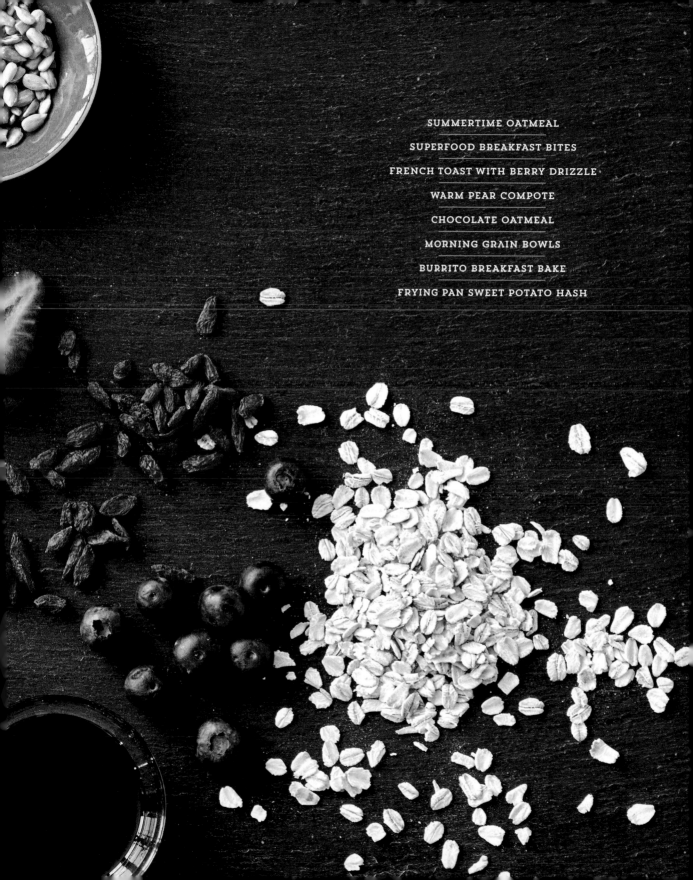

SUMMERTIME OATMEAL

SUPERFOOD BREAKFAST BITES

FRENCH TOAST WITH BERRY DRIZZLE

WARM PEAR COMPOTE

CHOCOLATE OATMEAL

MORNING GRAIN BOWLS

BURRITO BREAKFAST BAKE

FRYING PAN SWEET POTATO HASH

SUMMERTIME OATMEAL

MAKES: *2* SERVINGS · DIFFICULTY: *easy*

Some people think of oats as a hot cereal perfect for when leaves start falling or there's snow on the ground, but I love them all year round. In our house, we call this version Summertime Oatmeal because it's a cool and refreshing way to enjoy oatmeal even when it's sweltering outside. Prepare it the night before and spoon the goodness into jars for a quick and easy breakfast.

1 cup/100g rolled oats

1 tablespoon chia seeds

1 tablespoon ground flaxseeds (or linseeds)

½ teaspoon ground cinnamon

1¾ cups /425ml Almond Milk (page 2)

2 tablespoons Date Syrup (page 3)

1 2- to 3-inch/5 to 8cm piece vanilla pod, split and scraped (or 1 teaspoon extract)

⅔ cup/65g fresh or frozen blueberries or ⅔ cup/125g strawberries

Combine all the ingredients in a medium bowl and stir to mix. Spoon into two 1-pint/470ml jars with tight-fitting lids or two small bowls and cover tightly. Refrigerate overnight and remove the vanilla pod before serving.

MAXIMIZING YOUR MORNING

Want to start your day with a five-check mark breakfast? Add berries, flaxseeds, nuts and spices to your oatmeal. How about a six-plus-check mark smoothie? Create a thirst-quenching beverage by blending berries and other fruits, greens, flaxseeds and spices. (See pages 210 and 216.)

Daily Dozen Foods

✗ BERRIES   ✗ OTHER FRUITS   ✗ NUTS AND SEEDS   ✗ WHOLE GRAINS

SUPERFOOD BREAKFAST BITES

MAKES: *24* (1-INCH/2.5CM) BITES (4 TO 6 SERVINGS) · DIFFICULTY: *easy*

Stash these delicious bites in the fridge for an easy on-the-go breakfast or after-workout snack.

¾ cup /130g pitted dates, soaked in hot water for 20 minutes, then drained

¾ cup/185g raw walnuts, pecans or cashews

¾ cup/115g dried cranberries, apricots, apple slices or other dried fruit, chopped if necessary

¼ cup/35g sunflower seeds

2 tablespoons goji berries or barberries

2 tablespoons chia seeds or hemp hearts (hulled hemp seeds)

2 tablespoons ground flaxseeds (or linseeds)

1 1- to 1½-inch/2.5 to 4cm piece vanilla pod, split and scraped (or ½ teaspoon extract)

¼ teaspoon ground cinnamon

In a food processor, combine the drained dates and nuts and pulse until the nuts are finely ground and the dates are incorporated. Add the remaining ingredients and process until well combined. The mixture should be very sticky. If it seems too dry to hold together, add a little water, 1 tablespoon at a time. If the mixture is too wet, add a little more ground flaxseeds or some rolled oats.

Roll a heaped tablespoonful of the mixture between the palms of your hands to form a 1-inch/2.5cm ball. Transfer to a plate. Repeat until all the mixture has been rolled into balls. Cover the plate with foil or baking parchment and refrigerate for 4 hours before enjoying. Store in the refrigerator.

FLAXSEEDS

According to one remarkable study, flaxseeds (or linseeds) 'induced one of the most potent blood-pressure-lowering effects ever achieved by a dietary intervention.'[104] Eating just a few tablespoons a day appears to be two to three times more effective at lowering blood pressure than adopting an aerobic endurance exercise program[105] (not that you shouldn't do both!). Another study found that sprinkling a few spoonfuls of ground flaxseeds on your meals may reduce the risk of breast cancer.[106]

Daily Dozen Foods

X BERRIES   X OTHER FRUITS   X FLAXSEEDS   X NUTS AND SEEDS   X HERBS AND SPICES

FRENCH TOAST
WITH BERRY DRIZZLE

MAKES: *4* SERVINGS · DIFFICULTY: *easy*

The turmeric gives a warm golden color to this festive breakfast that packs six of the Daily Dozen in one dish.

BERRY DRIZZLE

1 cup/125g fresh or thawed frozen berries of choice

1 to 2 tablespoons Date Syrup (page 3)

FRENCH TOAST

1¼ cups/285ml Almond Milk (page 2)

2 tablespoons ground flaxseeds (or linseeds) blended with ¼ cup/60ml warm water

1 tablespoon date sugar

1 1- to 1½-inch/2.5 to 4cm piece vanilla pod, split and scraped (or ½ teaspoon extract)

1 ¼-inch/5mm piece fresh turmeric, grated (or ¼ teaspoon ground)

¼ teaspoon ground cinnamon

8 slices salt-free 100% whole-grain bread

BERRY DRIZZLE: Combine the berries and Date Syrup in a blender and blend until smooth. Transfer to a small jug or bowl and set aside.

FRENCH TOAST: In a blender, combine the Almond Milk, flax mixture, date sugar, vanilla, turmeric and cinnamon. Blend until well mixed. Transfer the batter to a shallow bowl. Heat a nonstick frying pan or griddle over medium-high heat. Working in batches, dip the bread slices into the batter, coating both sides, then place in the hot pan, and cook until golden brown on each side, turning once. Keep the cooked French toast warm in the oven set to its lowest temperature while you finish cooking the rest. When ready to serve, arrange the French toast on plates and drizzle with the berry syrup.

Daily Dozen Foods

✗ BERRIES ✗ OTHER FRUITS ✗ FLAXSEEDS ✗ NUTS AND SEEDS ✗ HERBS AND SPICES ✗ WHOLE GRAINS

WARM PEAR COMPOTE

MAKES: *4* SERVINGS · DIFFICULTY: *easy*

This delightful compote is a savory dessert or snack, as well as an incredible topping for oatmeal, French toast or pancakes.

2 tablespoons date sugar

2 teaspoons blended peeled lemon (see page 3)

2 tablespoons raisins

1 2- to 3-inch/5 to 8cm piece vanilla pod, split and scraped (or 1 teaspoon extract)

1 teaspoon ground cinnamon

¼ teaspoon ground ginger

⅛ teaspoon ground nutmeg

1 1-inch/2.5cm piece fresh turmeric, grated (or ⅛ teaspoon ground)

4 to 5 ripe Williams pears, cored and cut into bite-sized pieces

In a saucepan, combine ½ cup/120ml of water with all the ingredients, except the pears, and stir. Once blended, add the pear pieces and simmer over low heat until the pears are tender and the sauce has reduced, 15 to 20 minutes. Serve warm.

VARIATION: Use chopped apples, peaches or plums instead of pears.

Daily Dozen Foods

✗ OTHER FRUITS ✗ HERBS AND SPICES

CHOCOLATE OATMEAL

MAKES: *4* SERVINGS · DIFFICULTY: *easy*

Get creative with this recipe! Mix and match your favorite toppings, such as fresh berries and other fruits, chopped nuts or swirls of almond butter or peanut butter.

1½ cups/150g rolled oats

3 to 4 tablespoons unsweetened cocoa powder

½ teaspoon ground cinnamon

2 tablespoons chopped dried figs, goji berries or barberries

1 tablespoon ground flaxseeds (or linseeds)

1 tablespoon pumpkin seeds

2 tablespoons raisins (optional)

2 tablespoons Date Syrup (page 3)

In a saucepan, bring 3 cups/710ml of water to a boil and then stir in the oats, cocoa powder and cinnamon. Reduce the heat to low, add the figs, cover, and simmer for 5 minutes, stirring occasionally. Remove from the heat. Stir in the flaxseeds and pumpkin seeds. Cover and let stand for 2 minutes. To serve, spoon the oatmeal into bowls and top with the raisins (if using) and Date Syrup.

Daily Dozen Foods

✗ BERRIES   ✗ OTHER FRUITS   ✗ FLAXSEEDS   ✗ NUTS AND SEEDS   ✗ HERBS AND SPICES   ✗ WHOLE

MORNING GRAIN BOWLS

MAKES: *4* SERVINGS · DIFFICULTY: *easy*

Leftover cooked grains are a great way to start the day – and quick, too! If you don't have leftover grains, cook up a pot of your favorite grain the day before and you'll have the start of something good in the morning.

3 cups/480g cooked whole grains (brown rice, quinoa, freekeh or oats)

¾ cup/50g cooked cannellini beans, mashed

2 cups/500ml Almond Milk (page 2)

3 tablespoons ground flaxseeds (or linseeds)

1 1-inch/2.5cm piece fresh turmeric, grated (or 1 teaspoon ground)

1 teaspoon grated fresh ginger (optional)

1 cup/125g fresh or thawed frozen mixed berries

1 ripe banana, peeled and sliced

4 tablespoons Date Syrup (page 3) (optional)

In a microwave-safe bowl, combine the cooked grains, beans, Almond Milk, flaxseeds, turmeric and ginger (if using). Mix well. Microwave for 2 to 3 minutes, or until warm but not too hot. Divide the grain mixture among four bowls. Top each serving with about ¼ cup/30g of the berries and one-quarter of the sliced banana. Drizzle each serving with 1 tablespoon of Date Syrup, if desired.

BURRITO BREAKFAST BAKE

MAKES: *4* SERVINGS · DIFFICULTY: *moderate*

Baked sweet potatoes are one of my favorites – whether eaten as-is, spiced and seasoned, or featured in a dish like this one. To save time, I like to bake extras and keep them on hand or, in a pinch, quickly 'bake' one in the microwave.

½ cup/75g chopped red onion

1 orange or red pepper, finely chopped

6 cups/1.35kg chopped spinach, red chard or red kale

1 teaspoon Savory Spice Blend (page 4)

1 teaspoon chilli powder

½ teaspoon ground cumin

½ teaspoon dried oregano

2 cups/500g Summer Salsa (page 41) or your favorite salt-free salsa

1½ cups/95g cooked or 1 15.5-ounce/425g BPA-free tin or Tetra Pak* salt-free black beans, drained and rinsed

1 baked sweet potato, mashed

2 tablespoons minced fresh coriander

2 tablespoons nutritional yeast (or yeast flakes)

4 salt-free 100% whole-grain tortillas

¼ cup/30g coarsely ground pumpkin seeds

1 ripe Hass avocado, diced (optional)

1 fresh jalapeño pepper, chopped (optional)

Preheat the oven to 350°F/180°C/gas mark 4.

Combine the onion and pepper in a large saucepan with ¼ cup/60ml of water over medium heat. Cook for 5 minutes to soften. Add the greens, stirring until wilted and the water is evaporated. Add the Savory Spice Blend, chilli powder, cumin, oregano and ¼ cup/62g of the Summer Salsa, stirring to combine. Remove from the heat.

Mash the black beans in a large bowl. Add the reserved vegetable mixture and stir to mix well.

In a separate bowl, combine the mashed sweet potato, coriander, nutritional yeast and ¼ cup/62g of the salsa.

Spoon ¾ cup/190g of the salsa into a 9 × 13-inch/23 x 32cm baking dish, spreading evenly. Set aside.

Spoon one-quarter of the sweet potato mixture down the center of each tortilla. Top each with one-quarter of the bean mixture. Roll up the tortillas and arrange them, seam side down, in the prepared baking dish. Spread the remaining ¾ cup/190g of salsa over the burritos. Sprinkle with the pumpkin seeds. Cover and bake for 20 to 30 minutes, or until hot. Serve hot, garnished with diced avocado and chopped jalapeño, if desired.

* Tetra Pak is a type of aseptic packaging, meaning free from contamination from bacteria and other microorganisms, so the foods have very long shelf lives.

Daily Dozen Foods

✗ BEANS   ✗ GREENS   ✗ OTHER VEGETABLES   ✗ NUTS AND SEEDS   ✗ HERBS AND SPICES   ✗ WHOLE GRAINS

FRYING PAN SWEET POTATO HASH

MAKES: *4* SERVINGS · DIFFICULTY: *easy*

Although this recipe is in the Breakfast chapter, it's a rousing hit any time of the day or night. Make your Savory Spice Blend and Umami Sauce in advance to really cut down on the time it takes to prepare this dish. Can we talk spice? I love spicy foods, but know some people don't, so feel free to omit the cayenne. On the other hand, if you want even more heat, don't be shy about adding some Healthy Hot Sauce (page 8) when serving.

1 medium sweet potato, peeled and chopped

2 cups/650g chopped cauliflower

1 small red onion, chopped

1 red pepper, chopped

8 ounces/225g mushrooms, coarsely chopped

1½ cups/95g cooked or 1 15.5 ounce/425g BPA-free tin or Tetra Pak salt-free black or red beans, drained and rinsed

2 to 3 teaspoons Savory Spice Blend (page 4)

¼ teaspoon cayenne pepper or chilli flakes, or to taste

3 to 4 tablespoons Umami Sauce (page 5)

Preheat the oven to 425ºF/220ºC/gas mark 7 and line a baking sheet with a silicone mat or baking parchment. Spread the sweet potato on the prepared baking sheet and roast for 10 minutes; then add the cauliflower to the pan. Continue to roast until the sweet potatoes and cauliflower are tender, about 20 minutes. Remove from the oven and set aside.

Heat 2 tablespoons of water in a large frying pan over medium heat. Add the onion, cover, and cook until tender, about 5 minutes. Add the pepper and mushrooms and cook, uncovered, stirring until tender, about 5 minutes. Add the beans, Savory Spice Blend, cayenne and roasted vegetables and cook until heated through, about 5 minutes longer. Mash the ingredients lightly with a spatula, if desired. Drizzle with the Umami Sauce and serve hot.

VARIATION: Mix it up with different veggies. Instead of cauliflower, why not try courgette or another vegetable of your choosing?

Daily Dozen Foods

✗ BEANS ✗ CRUCIFEROUS VEGETABLES ✗ OTHER VEGETABLES ✗ HERBS AND SPICES

ARTICHOKE-SPINACH DIP

LEMONY HUMMUS

THREE-SEED CRACKERS

PUMPKIN SEED DIP

BLACK-EYED PEAS &
ROASTED RED PEPPER DIP

EDAMAME GUACAMOLE

SUMMER SALSA

CHEESY KALE CRISPS

SMOKY ROASTED CHICKPEAS

SNACKS, DIPS AND SPREADS

The recipes in this chapter are some of my all-time favorites when I'm feeling a little peckish and want a light lunch or a between-meal snack. When I'm on the road (or in the air), I often take some Cheesy Kale Crisps or Smoky Roasted Chickpeas with me. If you haven't noticed, convenience is almost as important to me as healthy (and flavorful) eating, which is why I really love the dips and spreads in this section. Each one can be enjoyed spread on Three-Seed Crackers or whole-grain bread, or served with raw veggies.

ARTICHOKE-SPINACH DIP

MAKES: *6* SERVINGS · DIFFICULTY: *easy*

Artichokes are remarkably high in antioxidants. I consider them too much of a pain to cook from scratch, so artichoke hearts are frequently included on my shopping list. They blend well with so many things, including spinach.

9 to 10 ounces/250 to 300g fresh or thawed frozen spinach, cooked and cooled

1 cup/62g cooked white beans, drained and rinsed

2 tablespoons nutritional yeast (or yeast flakes)

2 tablespoons minced spring onions

1 garlic clove, minced

2 teaspoons blended peeled lemon (see page 3)

2 teaspoons white miso paste

¼ teaspoon ground black pepper

Savory Spice Blend (page 4)

1 14-ounce/400g jar artichoke hearts, drained, or 1 10-ounce/300g packet frozen artichokes, cooked and cooled

Three-Seed Crackers (page 34), whole-grain crostini or crackers or raw veggies, to serve

Preheat the oven to 350°F/180°C/gas mark 4. Squeeze out the excess moisture from the cooled spinach and set aside. In a food processor, combine 2 tablespoons of water and the white beans, spring onions, garlic, lemon, miso paste, black pepper and Savory Spice Blend to taste and process until smooth and well blended. For a creamier texture, add a little more water, 1 tablespoon at a time. Add the artichokes and pulse until they are chopped. Add the spinach and pulse to combine. Transfer to a baking dish and bake until warm, 12 to 15 minutes. Spoon onto crackers or crostini, or serve as a dip for raw veggies.

VARIATION: Thin with some Almond Milk (page 2) or Vegetable Broth (page 6) and use as a sauce for pasta.

A CULINARY EXPLORER

Expand your culinary horizons beyond the many ways we already typically enjoy dips and spreads. Why not include one (or more) in a spring greens wrap? In the mood for pasta? Thin your favorite dip or spread with Almond Milk (page 2) or Vegetable Broth (page 6) and toss with cooked whole-grain pasta. You can even mix a dip or spread with grains and use it as a delicious stuffing for peppers and other veggies. The sky's the limit when it comes to thinking of different ways to incorporate these recipes into your menus.

Daily Dozen Foods

X BEANS   X GREENS   X OTHER VEGETABLES   X HERBS AND SPICES

LEMONY HUMMUS

MAKES: ABOUT *2* CUPS/450G · DIFFICULTY: *easy*

It's no secret that hummus is a wonderful dip for raw vegetables and a fantastic spread for spring greens wraps and other sandwiches . . . but did you know it even tastes great on whole-grain spaghetti? (I admit I've not only put hummus directly on pasta, but I've devoured it!)

2 garlic cloves, crushed

1 tablespoon blended peeled lemon (see page 3)

¼ cup/56g tahini

1 teaspoon white miso paste

1½ cups/255g cooked or 1 15.5-ounce/425g BPA-free tin or Tetra Pak salt-free chickpeas, drained and rinsed

¼ teaspoon ground cumin

¼ teaspoon smoked paprika

2 tablespoons chopped fresh parsley

In a food processor, combine the garlic and lemon and process until smooth. Add the tahini and miso paste and process once more until smooth. Add the chickpeas, cumin and paprika and process for several minutes until very smooth. Add a little water, 1 tablespoon at a time, if a thinner texture is desired. Taste and adjust the seasoning with more lemon or cumin, if needed. To serve, transfer to a bowl and sprinkle with the parsley.

VARIATIONS: Try any or all of these substitutions: replace the chickpeas with black beans or white beans, the parsley with coriander or dill, and the lemon with lime.

BPA

BPA, which stands for bisphenol A, is an industrial chemical that has been used since the 1950s in various plastic containers and the inside of many metal products, including tinned foods. Research has shown that BPA can seep into foods, causing possible negative health effects on the brain and/or heart, and may be linked to diabetes and obesity as well. More research is being undertaken to study BPA, but at the present time there are no federal restrictions on its use in food containers.

What to do? Many companies now make BPA-free containers – these should be clearly labeled. You might also consider using nonplastic or metal containers, such as glass or stainless steel.

Daily Dozen Foods

Ⅹ BEANS   Ⅹ NUTS AND SEEDS   Ⅹ HERBS AND SPICES

THREE-SEED CRACKERS

MAKES: ABOUT *25* (2¼-INCH/5.5CM) SQUARE CRACKERS · DIFFICULTY: *moderate*

Making your own crackers is easier (and more fun) than you might think. As a bonus, you can customize them to suit your taste, adding different seasonings as desired.

½ cup/65g raw pumpkin seeds

½ cup/65g raw sunflower seeds

½ cup/76g sesame seeds

1 ¼-inch/5mm piece fresh turmeric, grated (or ¼ teaspoon ground)

¼ cup/40g ground flaxseeds (or linseeds)

2 tablespoons minced fresh parsley

1 tablespoon nutritional yeast (or yeast flakes)

1½ teaspoons white miso paste

¼ teaspoon onion powder

1 teaspoon dried basil, dill, oregano or thyme (optional)

Preheat the oven to 250°F/120°C/gas mark ½. In a blender or food processor, grind the pumpkin seeds, sunflower seeds, ¼ cup/38g of the sesame seeds and the turmeric into a powder. Add the remaining ingredients, except the remaining sesame seeds, and pulse to combine and mix into a dough. If the dough is too dry, add up to 1 cup/250ml of water, 1 tablespoon at a time.

Spread out the dough flat on a baking sheet lined with a silicone mat or baking parchment. Top with another piece of baking parchment and roll out the dough evenly and thinly with a rolling pin or by pressing with your hands. (The rolled-out dough should be approximately a 12 × 10-inch/30 x 25cm rectangle.) Remove the top layer of baking parchment. Sprinkle with the remaining ¼ cup/38g of sesame seeds and lightly press them into the cracker dough. Use a sharp knife to score the crackers into the size you desire. Bake until lightly browned, about 3 hours. (For a crisper cracker, leave them in the oven with the heat turned off for a while longer.) Once cooled completely, the crackers may be stored at room temperature in a tightly covered container.

10 WAYS TO USE FLAXSEEDS (OR LINSEEDS)

Whether you buy flaxseeds preground or grind them at home in a spice grinder, coffee grinder or blender, you can enjoy this nutty superfood in all sorts of ways.

Here are a handful to get you started:

1. Sprinkle into oatmeal.
2. Shake onto salads.
3. Add to smoothies.
4. Use as a binder in burgers (pages 88 and 98) and loaves (page 156).
5. Add to homemade crackers (see above).
6. Use in your homemade energy bites (page 15).
7. Sprinkle on soups.
8. Use as a binder in baked goods.
9. Sprinkle on grain dishes.
10. Use as a thickener in sauces.

Daily Dozen Foods

✗ FLAXSEEDS ✗ NUTS AND SEEDS ✗ HERBS AND SPICES

PUMPKIN SEED DIP

MAKES: *3* CUPS/675G · DIFFICULTY: *easy*

Pumpkin seeds! They are delicious, nutritious and one of the most concentrated sources of zinc. Here's an interesting fact: Men need more zinc than women. Why? Because men lose zinc in every seminal emission. (Semen is filled with zinc.) In fact, men effectively lose about a quarter-cup's/30g's worth of pumpkin seeds every time! No matter your gender or (ahem) how much zinc you may want to replenish, enjoy this dip with raw veggies, as a spread for sandwiches, or thin out and use as sauce for pasta.

1¼ cups/160g raw unsalted pumpkin seeds

3 cloves Roasted Garlic (page 6)

1½ cups/95g cooked or 1 15.5-ounce/425g BPA-free tin or Tetra Pak salt free cannellini beans, drained and rinsed

1 teaspoon minced jalapeño pepper, or to taste (optional)

1 tablespoon tahini or almond butter

2 tablespoons blended peeled lemon (see page 3)

1½ teaspoons white miso paste

1 teaspoon Savory Spice Blend (page 4)

½ teaspoon smoked paprika

3 tablespoons minced fresh coriander (optional)

Assorted cut raw vegetables, for dipping

Preheat the oven to 250°F/120°C/gas mark ½. Line a baking sheet with a silicone mat or baking parchment. Spread the pumpkin seeds on the prepared baking sheet and toast for 15 to 18 minutes, or until they begin to lightly brown, stirring occasionally so they don't burn. Remove from the oven and set aside to cool.

Once the pumpkin seeds are cool to the touch, transfer them to a food processor and add the Roasted Garlic, beans, jalapeño (if using), tahini, lemon, miso, Savory Spice Blend, paprika and 3 tablespoons of water. Process until smooth. Transfer to a bowl and sprinkle with coriander, if desired. Serve with your favorite raw vegetable dippers.

Daily Dozen Foods

✗ BEANS   ✗ OTHER VEGETABLES   ✗ NUTS AND SEEDS   ✗ HERBS AND SPICES

BLACK-EYED PEAS & ROASTED RED PEPPER DIP

MAKES: ABOUT *3* CUPS/675G · DIFFICULTY: *easy*

Black-eyed peas are as marvelously nutritious as all the other legumes. They can be found frozen, tinned or dried at your local supermarket.

2 roasted red peppers (see page 9), or 1 9-ounce/250g jar roasted red peppers, drained

1½ cups/95g cooked or 1 15.5-ounce/425g BPA-free tin or Tetra Pak salt-free black-eyed peas, drained and rinsed

2 garlic cloves, crushed

1 teaspoon minced jalapeño pepper, or to taste

3 tablespoons tahini

1 tablespoon blended peeled lemon (see page 3)

1 teaspoon Savory Spice Blend (page 4)

1 teaspoon white miso paste

1 teaspoon smoked paprika

Cut raw vegetables, for dipping

In a food processor, combine the roasted red peppers, black-eyed peas, garlic and jalapeño and pulse to combine. Add the tahini, lemon, Savory Spice Blend, miso and paprika and process until smooth. Transfer the dip to a bowl and serve with the raw vegetable dippers.

VARIATIONS: Serve with toasted corn tortillas, or use as a spread for sandwiches or spring greens wraps.

Daily Dozen Foods

✗ BEANS   ✗ OTHER VEGETABLES   ✗ NUTS AND SEEDS   ✗ HERBS AND SPICES

EDAMAME GUACAMOLE

MAKES: ABOUT 1½ CUPS/335G · DIFFICULTY: *easy*

Edamame has been a long-time favorite snack of mine. They're so good I can eat a seemingly endless amount of them right from their pods. This recipe calls for them to be incorporated into a creative take on guacamole, which I love just as much as enjoying them au naturel.

The problem with guacamole is that most people want to dip salted, deep-fried tortilla chips into it. Don't do it! Skip the chip in favor of raw vegetables, such as carrots or pepper strips. Or, do as I do, and dip with steamed asparagus.

1 cup/75g frozen shelled edamame, thawed

1 ripe Hass avocado, peeled and pitted

2 teaspoons blended peeled lime (see page 3)

1 teaspoon Savory Spice Blend (page 4)

⅛ to ¼ teaspoon ground cumin, or to taste

1 Roma tomato, finely chopped

2 tablespoons chopped fresh coriander

1 tablespoon minced red onion

1 tablespoon minced jalapeño pepper (optional)

Steamed asparagus or raw vegetables, for dipping

Cook the edamame in a saucepan of boiling water until tender, 10 to 12 minutes. Drain and set aside to cool.

In a food processor, combine the edamame, avocado, lime, Savory Spice Blend and cumin, and process until smooth. Transfer to a bowl and fold in the tomato, coriander, onion and jalapeño (if using). Serve with vegetables for dipping.

Daily Dozen Foods

✗ BEANS   ✗ OTHER FRUITS   ✗ OTHER VEGETABLES   ✗ HERBS AND SPICES

SUMMER SALSA

MAKES: ABOUT *3* CUPS/675G · DIFFICULTY: *easy*

Homemade salsa is best when fresh tomatoes are at their peak. One of my favorite things about making my own salsa is that I can really make it special. Depending on what I'm craving in the moment, I can add as much or as little heat, double or outright skip the coriander, add such veggies as corn, carrots, and whatever else may tickle my fancy (and my taste buds).

---

6 firm plum tomatoes, cored and coarsely chopped

½ orange or yellow pepper, minced

2 tablespoons minced red onion

1 jalapeño or other small hot chilli pepper, seeded and minced

2 teaspoons blended peeled lime (see page 3)

2 tablespoons minced fresh coriander

2 tablespoons minced fresh parsley

Savory Spice Blend (page 4)

In a bowl, combine all the ingredients, adding Savory Spice Blend to taste, and stir well. Cover and let stand at room temperature for 1 hour before serving. If not using right away, store in the refrigerator. The salsa will keep refrigerated for 3 to 4 days.

FRUIT

Although each recipe in this chapter makes a healthy snack, don't forget that nature's best snack food is fruit. Abundant, inexpensive and healthy, fruit satisfies your midday hunger and tastes great as well. Anyone who thinks it's not convenient to eat plant-based has never met an apple.

Daily Dozen Foods

✗ OTHER VEGETABLES   ✗ HERBS AND SPICES

CHEESY KALE CRISPS

MAKES: *4* SERVINGS · DIFFICULTY: *moderate*

What a great way to eat your greens! Kale, one of the oldest forms of cultivated cabbage, is easy to grow and filled with such dark green leafy goodness. My dear friend Essy (Dr. Caldwell Esselstyn Jr.) eats as much of it and other dark green leafies as he can throughout the day. You'll be seeing kale in many of the recipes in this book – for good reason!

1 bunch red kale, thick stems removed

½ cup/75g raw cashews, soaked for 3 hours and then drained

½ cup/85g roasted red pepper (see page 9), or shop-bought

3 tablespoons nutritional yeast (or yeast flakes)

1 teaspoon rice vinegar

1 teaspoon white miso paste

1 ¼-inch/5mm piece fresh turmeric, grated (or ¼ teaspoon ground)

1 teaspoon smoked paprika

Wash the kale leaves well and then tear or cut any large leaves into 2-inch/5cm pieces. Dry the kale pieces in a salad spinner or a clean tea towel. Once the kale is very dry, transfer it to a large bowl and set aside. Preheat the oven to 350°F/180°C/gas mark 4. Line two large baking sheets with silicone mats and set aside.

In a food processor or high-speed blender, combine 2 tablespoons of water and the remaining ingredients and process until smooth. The sauce should be thick enough to coat the kale. If it's too thick, add a little more water, 1 tablespoon at a time. Pour the sauce onto the kale and toss to coat, massaging the sauce into the leaves. Arrange the kale in a single layer on the prepared baking sheets and bake for 20 minutes. Remove any pieces that are crisp and turn over any that have not yet crisped before returning the trays to the oven for 2 to 5 minutes longer, or until the remaining kale pieces are crisp. Be sure to watch so they don't burn. Set aside to cool completely before eating.

Daily Dozen Foods

✗ GREENS   ✗ OTHER VEGETABLES   ✗ NUTS AND SEEDS   ✗ HERBS AND SPICES

SMOKY ROASTED CHICKPEAS

MAKES ABOUT *1½* CUPS/255G · DIFFICULTY: *easy*

More chickpeas! There are just so many things you can do with these little protein- and fiber-packed legumes. I can't get enough of them, and neither should you!

1½ cups/255g cooked or 1 15.5-ounce /425g BPA-free tin or Tetra Pak salt-free chickpeas, drained, well rinsed and blotted dry

1 tablespoon Date Syrup (page 3)

1 tablespoon nutritional yeast (or yeast flakes)

2 teaspoons white miso paste

1½ teaspoons smoked paprika

¼ teaspoon onion powder

½ teaspoon Savory Spice Blend (page 4)

Preheat the oven to 375°F/190°C/gas mark 5. Line a baking sheet with a silicone mat or baking parchment and set aside. Make sure the chickpeas are as dry as possible and remove any loose skins.

In a medium bowl, combine 2 tablespoons of water and all the remaining ingredients, except the chickpeas and Savory Spice Blend. Add the chickpeas and toss to coat evenly.

Transfer the chickpeas to the prepared baking sheet, spreading evenly in a single layer. Bake for 30 to 35 minutes, stirring every 8 to 10 minutes, until lightly browned and crunchy. Sprinkle the roasted chickpeas with the spice blend and serve warm or at room temperature. These are best eaten on the day they are made.

POPCORN

One of my all-time favorite snacks is air-popped popcorn with nutritional yeast. If you aren't already familiar with it, nutritional yeast is a deactivated yeast (meaning it doesn't grow like baking yeast) and has a cheesy, nutty flavor (as opposed to brewer's yeast, a beer industry by-product that tastes nasty). I just wish it had a better name. Where was the person who came up with 'aquafaba' when nutritional yeast was being named? In New Zealand, it's called Brufax. I don't know if that's worse. Those in the know call it 'nooch'. Okay, that's pretty cute.

Daily Dozen Foods

✗ BEANS ✗ HERBS AND SPICES

SOUPS AND CHILLIES

Soups and chillies are the ultimate comfort food. Warming and satisfying, they are a wonderful way to incorporate so many delicious ingredients into a single dish. Start with the hearty bean and vegetable soups and expand your repertoire to Asian-inspired soups and savory chillies.

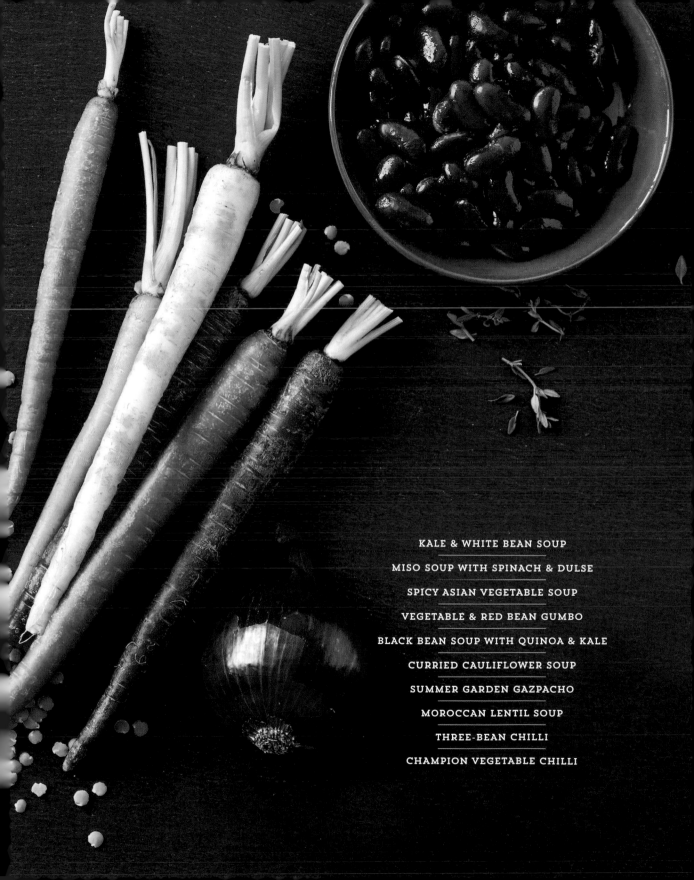

KALE & WHITE BEAN SOUP

MISO SOUP WITH SPINACH & DULSE

SPICY ASIAN VEGETABLE SOUP

VEGETABLE & RED BEAN GUMBO

BLACK BEAN SOUP WITH QUINOA & KALE

CURRIED CAULIFLOWER SOUP

SUMMER GARDEN GAZPACHO

MOROCCAN LENTIL SOUP

THREE-BEAN CHILLI

CHAMPION VEGETABLE CHILLI

KALE & WHITE BEAN SOUP

MAKES: *4* SERVINGS · DIFFICULTY: *easy*

Kale, kale, and more kale! I can't seem to get enough of it, but if you'd like, feel free to substitute a different variety of greens in this recipe. I think Swiss chard would be delicious!

6 cups/1.4 liters Vegetable Broth (page 6)

1 large red onion, chopped

3 to 4 garlic cloves, minced

1 medium sweet potato, cut into ½-inch/1cm dice

5 cups /350g chopped fresh red kale

¼ teaspoon chilli flakes (or more . . . much, much more, if you love spice as I do)

2 bay leaves

1½ cups/95g cooked or 1 15.5-ounce/425g BPA-free tin or Tetra Pak salt-free cannellini beans, drained and rinsed

1 teaspoon white miso paste

2 tablespoons nutritional yeast (or yeast flakes)

2 tablespoons chopped fresh parsley

1 teaspoon fresh marjoram or oregano, or ½ teaspoon dried

2 teaspoons Savory Spice Blend (page 4), or to taste

Heat 1 cup/250ml of the broth in a large pan over medium heat. Add the onion and garlic and simmer for 5 minutes. Stir in the sweet potato, kale, chilli flakes, bay leaves and the remaining 5 cups/1.2 liters of broth and bring to a boil over high heat. Lower the heat to medium, add the beans, and cook until the vegetables are tender, 20 to 30 minutes. Ladle about ⅓ cup/80ml of the broth into a small bowl or cup. Add the miso paste and stir to blend. Pour the miso mixture into the soup and stir in the nutritional yeast, parsley, marjoram and Savory Spice Blend. Serve hot.

Daily Dozen Foods

✗ BEANS   ✗ GREENS   ✗ OTHER VEGETABLES   ✗ HERBS AND SPICES

MISO SOUP WITH SPINACH & DULSE

MAKES: *4* SERVINGS · DIFFICULTY: *easy*

One of the milder-tasting seaweeds, dried dulse is a good gateway plant to the world of sea vegetables, underwater dark green leafies. Seaweeds aren't just flavorful; they're rich with nutrients, including iodine, which is especially critical for pregnant women. I used to get regular doses of iodine from the Eden brand beans I favored, as the company tins its beans with a bit of seaweed called kombu. Since I started pressure-cooking my own beans, I've gotten into the habit of snacking on sheets of seaweed called nori. You can find nori in a variety of flavors with all sorts of seasonings. I used to play around and season my own, but I've taken to simply eating them straight. Two sheets a day should be all the iodine you need.

3 tablespoons dried dulse, soaked in water for 3 minutes, then drained

5 cups/1.2 liters Vegetable Broth (page 6)

1 cup/75g shelled edamame, fresh or thawed if frozen

6 shiitake mushroom caps, thinly sliced

3 spring onions, chopped

¼ cup/55g white miso paste

4 cups/900g fresh spinach, cut into strips

Savory Spice Blend (page 4)

Chop the dulse and set aside. Heat the broth in a large saucepan over high heat and bring to a boil. Add the edamame and lower the heat to medium. Simmer for 5 minutes, stir in the mushrooms and spring onions, and simmer for 5 minutes longer. Reduce the heat to low. In a small bowl, mix together the miso paste with about ⅓ cup/80ml of the hot broth, blending well. Add the blended miso mixture to the soup. Add the dulse, spinach and Savory Spice Blend to taste and simmer for about 3 minutes. Do not boil. Serve hot.

Daily Dozen Foods

✗ BEANS   ✗ GREENS   ✗ OTHER VEGETABLES   ✗ HERBS AND SPICES

SPICY ASIAN VEGETABLE SOUP

MAKES: *4* SERVINGS · DIFFICULTY: *easy*

For an even heartier version of this amazing soup, add cooked 100% buckwheat noodles or brown, black or red rice just before serving.

5 cups/1.2 liters Vegetable Broth (page 6)

1 4-inch/10cm piece lemongrass, crushed

4 tablespoons grated fresh ginger

1 garlic clove, minced

2 cups/150g sliced shiitake mushroom caps

2 shallots, cut lengthwise into thin slivers

2 cups/200g thinly sliced bok choy or chinese leaf

1 cup/150g shredded carrot

3 spring onions, chopped

2 teaspoons blended peeled lime (see page 3), or to taste

4 cherry tomatoes, halved

1 teaspoon Healthy Hot Sauce (page 8), or to taste

2 teaspoons Savory Spice Blend (page 4), or to taste

2 tablespoons chopped fresh Thai basil or coriander

In a large pan, combine the broth, lemongrass, ginger and garlic. Bring to a boil, then reduce the heat to low, cover, and simmer for 20 minutes. Remove the lemongrass and bring to a boil. Add the mushrooms, shallots, bok choy and carrot. Reduce the heat to low and cook for 3 minutes. Stir in the spring onions, lime, tomatoes, Healthy Hot Sauce and Savory Spice Blend. Simmer until hot, about 2 minutes. Garnish with Thai basil or coriander and serve hot.

Daily Dozen Foods

✗ CRUCIFEROUS VEGETABLES   ✗ OTHER VEGETABLES   ✗ HERBS AND SPICES

VEGETABLE & RED BEAN GUMBO

MAKES: *4* SERVINGS · DIFFICULTY: *easy*

Some people swear by okra, and others are more than happy to do without it. If you're not okra's biggest fan, skip it and just a dd more courgette or green beans to this rich stew. But okra is packed with cholesterol-lowering soluble fiber, so I encourage you to give it one more try before you give it a hard pass.

6 cups/1.4 liters Vegetable Broth (page 6) or water

1 medium red onion, chopped

1 green pepper, seeded and chopped

½ cup/50g celery, minced

2 or 3 garlic cloves, minced

1 14.5-ounce/400g BPA-free tin or Tetra Pak salt-free diced tomatoes, undrained

1½ cups/150g sliced okra, fresh or thawed if frozen

1 cup/175g diced courgette or cut green beans

3 teaspoons fresh thyme, or 1 teaspoon dried

1 teaspoon dried marjoram or oregano, or 3 teaspoons fresh

1 teaspoon smoked paprika

2 teaspoons salt-free Cajun seasoning (optional)

1½ cups/95g cooked or 1 15.5-ounce/425g BPA-free tin or Tetra Pak salt-free dark red kidney beans or black-eyed peas, drained and rinsed

½ teaspoon chilli flakes, or to taste

2 teaspoons Savory Spice Blend (page 4), or to taste

3 cups/750g cooked brown, black or red rice, to serve (see note)

Heat 1 cup/250ml of the broth in a large pan over medium-high heat. Add the onion, pepper, celery and garlic and cook for 5 minutes, stirring occasionally. Stir in the tomatoes with their juices, okra, courgette, thyme, marjoram, paprika and Cajun seasoning (if using). Add the remaining 5 cups/1.2 liters of broth and bring to a boil. Lower the heat to a simmer, stir in the beans, and cook until the vegetables are tender, 20 to 30 minutes. Stir in the chilli flakes and Savory Spice Blend. Serve hot in shallow bowls over the cooked rice.

NOTE: Due to recent studies on the arsenic content in rice, Dr. Greger now recommends diversifying your grains. Wherever a recipe calls for rice, please consider using other whole intake grains, such as quinoa, millet, oat groats, hulled (not pearled) barley, buckwheat or wheat berries.

Daily Dozen Foods

✗ BEANS ✗ OTHER VEGETABLES ✗ HERBS AND SPICES ✗ WHOLE GRAINS

SO MANY PLANTS...

To give you a sense of the variety of healthy foods out there, let me tell you a funny story about the love of my life, Andrea. (Bet you thought I was going to say kale!) When we were first dating ages ago and friends would ask me what she was like, I'd share this with them, as I felt it best summed up her joie de vivre: Andrea decided early on that life was too short to eat the same meal twice. And I mean, *ever*. This was just part of her perpetual seize-the-day attitude, and it continues today. Every week, she pulls out cookbooks and charts out new recipes for each main meal, making sure to pencil in a notation at the bottom of each so she doesn't forget and accidentally make the same dish some years in the future. The most endearing part is that she thinks everyone else is weird for not sharing her passion for culinary adventure.

Of course, cooking for her became a challenge. Whenever I made something I really liked, it came with a degree of sadness, because I knew we'd never be able to have that dish again. (Although one time I was able to sneak in a repeat performance of my tried-and-true Green Light Mac & Cheese (page 143) by disguising it with enough blended spinach to turn it bright green, and she was none the wiser. Shhh!) The good news is there are so many wonderful whole-plant foods that Andrea can maintain her never-repeat-a-meal habit for the rest of her long, long life.

BLACK BEAN SOUP WITH QUINOA & KALE

MAKES: *4* SERVINGS · DIFFICULTY: *easy*

Quinoa is a relatively new addition to my diet. I had been looking for different whole grains I could add to my pantry and discovered this gem. When you're at the market, look for the colored varieties, such as red or black quinoa. In fact, I always look for color to get the added benefit of the antioxidant power of the plant pigments. So, I buy red or black rice rather than brown (and never white) and always pick red onions over white and red cabbage over green.

4 cups/950ml Vegetable Broth (page 6)

1 red onion, chopped

1 carrot, chopped

1 celery stalk, chopped

2 garlic cloves, minced

1 sweet potato, peeled and chopped

1 bay leaf

⅓ cup/55g quinoa, rinsed and drained

3 cups/185g cooked black beans or 2 15.5-ounce/425g BPA-free tins or Tetra Paks black beans, drained and rinsed

1 14.5-ounce/400g BPA-free tin or Tetra Pak diced, unsalted tomatoes, undrained

2 teaspoons Savory Spice Blend (page 4)

1 teaspoon ground cumin

½ teaspoon dried oregano

Ground black pepper, to taste

3 cups/200g chopped red kale

In a large pan, heat 1 cup/250ml of the broth over medium-high heat. Add the onion, carrot, celery, garlic and sweet potato. Cook, stirring occasionally, until the vegetables have softened, about 5 minutes. Add the bay leaf, quinoa, beans, tomatoes, Savory Spice Blend, herbs, black pepper and the remaining 3 cups/700ml of broth and bring to a boil. Lower the heat to a simmer and stir in the kale. Cover and cook until the quinoa and vegetables are tender, about 30 minutes. Remove and discard the bay leaf, and serve hot.

KALE

Researchers have found that kale may help control cholesterol levels. In one study, kale substantially lowered participants' bad (LDL) cholesterol and boosted their good (HDL) cholesterol[107] as much as running 300 miles.[108] Although it has been recently called into question whether raising HDL cholesterol actually makes a difference,[109] I still think kale is the bee's knees and well worthy of its nickname 'queen of greens'.

Daily Dozen Foods

X BEANS   X GREENS   X OTHER VEGETABLES   X HERBS AND SPICES   X WHOLE GRAINS

CURRIED CAULIFLOWER SOUP

MAKES: *4* SERVINGS · DIFFICULTY: *easy*

Cauliflower is one of two great exceptions to the white foods rule. Yes, I opt for color to take advantage of the antioxidant boost from plant pigments and shun refined grains, such as white bread and white rice, but although cauliflower might be white, just like its cruciferous cousins, it's one of the healthiest vegetables. (The other unusually healthy white food? White mushrooms.)

4 cups/950ml Vegetable Broth (page 6)

1 red onion, chopped

1 garlic clove, minced

1½ teaspoons grated fresh ginger

1½ tablespoons curry powder

2 teaspoons date sugar

1 teaspoon Savory Spice Blend (page 4)

1 head cauliflower, trimmed and coarsely chopped

2 teaspoons blended peeled lemon (see page 3)

1 plum tomato, finely chopped, for garnish

In a large pan, heat 1 cup/250ml of the broth over medium-high heat. Add the onion and cook until softened, about 5 minutes. Stir in the garlic, ginger, curry, date sugar and Savory Spice Blend. Add the cauliflower and the remaining 3 cups/700ml of broth and bring to a boil. Lower the heat to a simmer, cover, and cook until the cauliflower is soft, about 30 minutes.

Purée the soup in a food processor or blender, working in batches if necessary, or use a stick blender to purée the soup directly in the pan. Stir in the lemon; then taste and adjust the seasonings as desired. Ladle into bowls and serve hot, garnished with chopped tomato.

VARIATIONS: When ready to serve, add any of the following for a slightly different take on what will surely become a favorite: cooked brown, red or black rice; green peas; chopped cooked spinach; minced chives; or diced spring onions.

Daily Dozen Foods

X CRUCIFEROUS VEGETABLES   X OTHER VEGETABLES   X HERBS AND SPICES

SUMMER GARDEN GAZPACHO

MAKES: *4* SERVINGS · DIFFICULTY: *easy*

By adding cannellini beans to this refreshing gazpacho, you'll create a more satisfying soup.

2 large tomatoes, halved and cored

1 small red pepper, halved and seeded

¼ cup/38g coarsely chopped sweet red onion

1 cup/150g chopped cucumber

1 small yellow pepper, seeded and chopped

1 garlic clove, minced

1 chilli pepper, seeded and minced (and as spicy as you can handle)

2 tablespoons minced spring onion

3 tablespoons rice vinegar

1 teaspoon Healthy Hot Sauce (page 8) (optional)

2½ cups/600ml unsalted vegetable juice blend, such as V-12 Vegetable Blast (page 219)

¼ cup/4 tablespoons minced fresh parsley

1 ¼-inch/5mm piece fresh turmeric, grated (or ¼ teaspoon ground)

Savory Spice Blend (page 4)

1½ cups/95g cooked or 1 15.5-ounce/425g BPA-free tin or Tetra Pak salt-free cannellini beans, drained and rinsed (optional)

1 teaspoon blended peeled lemon (see page 3)

In a blender or food processor, combine the tomatoes, red pepper and onion and process until smooth. Pour the vegetable mixture into a large bowl and stir in the cucumber, yellow pepper, garlic, chilli and spring onions. Add the vinegar and Healthy Hot Sauce (if using), and stir in the vegetable juice blend, 2 tablespoons of the parsley, the turmeric and Savory Spice Blend to taste. Stir in the beans (if using). Cover the bowl and refrigerate at least 2 hours to chill and allow flavors to develop. Just before serving, stir in the lemon to brighten the flavors. Serve the soup chilled and garnished with the remaining parsley.

Daily Dozen Foods

✗ BEANS (OPTIONALLY)   ✗ OTHER VEGETABLES   ✗ HERBS AND SPICES

MOROCCAN LENTIL SOUP

MAKES: *4* SERVINGS · DIFFICULTY: *easy*

Lentils are my favorite legume. They cook so quickly, mix well with just about everything, and are exceptionally nutrient dense. I never prepare rice or other grains without throwing in some lentils. Don't forget that any dish can be made healthier by adding beans or greens. A variety of herbs and spices elevate this particular lentil soup from simple to sensational.

5 cups/1.2 liters Vegetable Broth (page 6) or water

1 red onion, chopped

2 garlic cloves, chopped

1 red pepper, chopped

1 teaspoon grated fresh ginger

1 teaspoon ground coriander

½ teaspoon ground cumin

½ teaspoon ground cinnamon

1 ¼-inch/5mm piece fresh turmeric, grated (or ¼ teaspoon ground)

¼ teaspoon chilli flakes

¼ teaspoon ground fennel seeds

1 cup/200g dried black or red lentils

1 14.5-ounce/400g BPA-free tin or Tetra Pak salt-free diced tomatoes, undrained

1 teaspoon Savory Spice Blend (page 4), or to taste

4 cups/400g chopped baby greens

In a large pan, heat 1 cup/250ml of the broth over medium heat. Add the onion, garlic and pepper. Cook until slightly softened, about 5 minutes. Add the ginger, coriander, cumin, cinnamon, turmeric, chilli flakes and fennel seeds; then stir in the lentils, tomatoes and remaining 4 cups/950ml of broth. Bring to a boil. Lower the heat to a simmer, cover, and cook until the lentils are soft, 15 to 20 minutes. Add the Savory Spice Blend and stir in the baby greens, simmering until wilted. Serve hot.

COOKING WITH SPICE

With all the exotic, exciting and excellent spices on the market, you have no excuse not to go out and experiment with new flavors. Myself, I have become very fond of smoked paprika. It's not as easy to find as regular paprika, so I order it online. As much as I love greens, greens with smoked paprika are even better. I'm also very fond of Ceylon cinnamon. I take packets of unsweetened cocoa powder and cinnamon whenever I travel, to make bad hotel coffee taste better. I am also a fan of black pepper. Not the most mysterious of spices, it's a favored staple for a reason. It's so good!

Cooking with spices means paying attention, though. I once made what became known in my family as cardamom death muffins. I was following a recipe for blueberry muffins that called for a bit of dried cardamom. As I prepared my batter, I used the right amount of cardamom, but fresh, not dried. Oh, *wow*, was that a mistake! The muffins were so overpowering that after just one bite, our eyes started watering. I would have figured the dried spice, being concentrated, would be more potent than fresh. Not so!

Daily Dozen Foods

X BEANS   X GREENS   X OTHER VEGETABLES   X HERBS AND SPICES

THREE-BEAN CHILLI

MAKES: *4* SERVINGS · DIFFICULTY: *easy*

Enjoy this tasty chilli alone or on a bed of brown, red or black rice or cooked greens (or both). It's also a great topping for sweet potatoes.

2 cups/500ml Vegetable Broth (page 6)

1 red onion, chopped

1 pepper (any color), seeded and chopped

2 garlic cloves, minced

1 small hot chilli pepper, seeded and minced

2 to 3 cups/200 to 300g chopped mushrooms

2 tablespoons chilli powder, or to taste

¼ cup/56g jarred tomato purée

1 14.5-ounce/400g BPA-free tin or Tetra Pak salt-free diced tomatoes, undrained

½ cup/100g dried red lentils

1½ cups/95g cooked or 1 15.5-ounce/425g BPA-free tin or Tetra Pak salt-free kidney beans, drained and rinsed

1½ cups/95g cooked or 1 15.5-ounce/425g BPA-free tin or Tetra Pak salt-free black beans, drained and rinsed

2 tablespoons Umami Sauce (page 5)

1 ¼-inch/5mm piece fresh turmeric, grated (or ¼ teaspoon ground)

1 tablespoon Savory Spice Blend (page 4), or to taste

½ teaspoon smoked paprika

¼ teaspoon ground black pepper

In a large pan, heat 1 cup/250ml of the broth over medium heat. Add the onion and pepper and cook until softened, stirring occasionally, about 5 minutes. Add the garlic, minced chilli, and mushrooms; then stir in the chilli powder and tomato purée. Add the remaining ingredients, including the second cup of broth, and simmer, stirring occasionally, until the lentils are tender and the flavors are blended, about 50 minutes. Taste to adjust the seasonings, if needed, and serve hot.

CHILLI VARIATIONS

Just as there are countless ways to make chilli, there are just as many ways to serve it. Try it on a bed of cooked greens or whole grains. Use it as a taco filling. Toss it with whole wheat pasta. Top baked sweet potatoes or winter squash with it. Experiment and enjoy!

Daily Dozen Foods

✗ BEANS   ✗ OTHER VEGETABLES   ✗ HERBS AND SPICES

CHAMPION VEGETABLE CHILLI

MAKES: *4* SERVINGS · DIFFICULTY: *easy*

Here's another excellent chilli variety that can be served in many ways. Try this over baked and mashed sweet potato; brown, black or red rice; quinoa; or greens greens greens. Use it as a filling in a spring greens wrap. Let us know what other creative ways you come up with to enjoy this dish!

1½ cups/360ml Vegetable Broth (page 6)

1 red onion, chopped

½ cup/50g minced celery

2 to 3 cups/200 to 300g chopped mushrooms (any kind)

1 red pepper, seeded and chopped

1 courgette, chopped

1 small hot chilli pepper, seeded and finely minced (optional)

2 garlic cloves, minced

3 tablespoons jarred tomato purée

2 tablespoons chilli powder, or to taste

1 ¼-inch/5mm piece fresh turmeric, grated (or ¼ teaspoon ground)

1 14.5-ounce/400g BPA-free tin or Tetra Pak salt-free diced tomatoes, undrained

3 cups/185g cooked or 2 15.5-ounce/425g BPA-free tins or Tetra Paks pinto beans, drained and rinsed

1 cup/175g corn kernels

2 teaspoons Savory Spice Blend (page 4), or to taste

½ teaspoon smoked paprika

In a large pan, heat 1 cup/250ml of the broth over medium heat. Add the onion and celery and cook until softened, about 5 minutes. Add the mushrooms, pepper, courgette, chilli (if using) and garlic and cook until softened, stirring occasionally, about 10 minutes. Stir in the tomato purée, chilli powder and turmeric; then add the tomatoes, pinto beans and remaining ½ cup/110ml of broth. Simmer until the vegetables are tender, stirring occasionally, about 45 minutes. Add a little water if the chilli gets too thick to your liking. Stir in the corn, Savory Spice Blend and paprika. Serve hot.

Daily Dozen Foods

✗ BEANS   ✗ OTHER VEGETABLES   ✗ HERBS AND SPICES

SALADS AND DRESSINGS

You won't find any recipes in this cookbook for a side salad of iceberg lettuce with a few carrot shavings and half a cherry tomato, mayonnaise-laden macaroni salad, or any other so-called salad that's virtually devoid of taste and nutrition. The salads in this chapter are rich with flavor and crunch, and can be served as your entrée, a starter, a side, or even a snack. And, with so much added goodness, including nuts, seeds and fruits, you'll keep busy ticking off lots of the Daily Dozen checkboxes.

GOLDEN QUINOA TABBOULEH

KALE SALAD WITH AVOCADO
GODDESS DRESSING

BLACK BEAN GAZPACHO SALAD

SESAME RED CABBAGE &
CARROT SLAW

CHOPPED VEGETABLE SALAD

MANGO-AVOCADO-KALE SALAD WITH
GINGER-SESAME ORANGE DRESSING

SUPER SALAD WITH GARLIC CAESAR
DRESSING & HEMP HEARTS

PISTACHIO-SPINACH SALAD WITH
STRAWBERRY BALSAMIC DRESSING

GOLDEN QUINOA TABBOULEH

MAKES: *6* SERVINGS · DIFFICULTY: *easy*

Turmeric adds a touch of gold to the quinoa in this tasty riff on tabbouleh. More than fifty clinical trials have tested turmeric against a variety of diseases, including lung and brain diseases and a variety of cancers. It's been shown to make colon polyps disappear, speed recovery after surgery, and treat rheumatoid arthritis better than the leading drug. Turmeric also appears to be effective in treating osteoarthritis and other inflammatory conditions, such as lupus and inflammatory bowel disease. I recommend a quarter-teaspoon a day.

1 cup/170g quinoa, washed well, rinsed and drained

1 ¼-inch/5mm piece fresh turmeric, grated (or ¼ teaspoon ground)

DRESSING

2 tablespoons blended peeled lemon (see page 3)

1 tablespoon Date Syrup (page 3)

1½ teaspoons Savory Spice Blend (page 4)

SALAD

1½ cups/255g cooked or 1 15.5-ounce/425g BPA-free tin or Tetra Pak salt-free chickpeas, drained and rinsed

2 Roma tomatoes, chopped

1 small ripe Hass avocado, peeled, pitted and diced

1 cup/150g chopped cucumber

½ cup/15g minced fresh parsley, mint or coriander

2 spring onions, minced

Ground black pepper

4 cups/300g torn salad greens (my favorite is baby rocket), to serve

In a saucepan, bring 1¾ cups/430ml of water to a boil. Add the quinoa and turmeric and reduce the heat to low. Cover and simmer until the water is absorbed, about 15 minutes. Drain well to remove any excess moisture. Transfer the quinoa to a large bowl and set aside to cool.

DRESSING: In a small bowl, combine the lemon, Date Syrup, Savory Spice Blend and 3 tablespoons of water.

SALAD: When the quinoa is cool, add the chickpeas, tomatoes, avocado, cucumber, parsley and spring onions. Pour on the dressing and season with black pepper to taste. Mix gently to combine. Cover and refrigerate for at least 1 hour, or until ready to serve. The tabbouleh tastes best if enjoyed on the same day it is made. To serve, spoon over torn salad greens.

10 WAYS TO GET YOUR DAILY TURMERIC

1. Add it to a smoothie.
2. Use it in curries (page 130).
3. Add it to grain dishes (page 140).
4. Blend it into salad dressings.
5. Add it to pasta dishes.
6. Mash it into a baked sweet potato.
7. Add it to soups.
8. Sprinkle it on your oatmeal.
9. Blend it into bean spreads.
10. Add it to your pumpkin pie.

Daily Dozen Foods

✗ BEANS   ✗ GREENS   ✗ OTHER VEGETABLES   ✗ HERBS AND SPICES   ✗ WHOLE GRAINS

KALE SALAD WITH AVOCADO GODDESS DRESSING

MAKES: *4* SERVINGS · DIFFICULTY: *easy*

Is there anything kale cannot do?

DRESSING

1 small ripe Hass avocado, peeled and pitted

1 spring onion, coarsely chopped

1 garlic clove, crushed

¼ cup/4 tablespoons chopped fresh parsley

1 tablespoon minced fresh tarragon, or 1 teaspoon dried

2 tablespoons rice vinegar

2 teaspoons blended peeled lemon (see page 3)

1 tablespoon nutritional yeast (or yeast flakes)

1 teaspoon Date Syrup (page 3)

½ teaspoon white miso paste

½ teaspoon Savory Spice Blend (page 4), or to taste

SALAD

4 small or medium beetroots, trimmed and scrubbed

1 bunch red kale, washed, tough stems removed

1½ cups/95g cooked or 1 15.5-ounce/425g BPA-free tin or Tetra Pak salt-free black beans, drained and rinsed

¼ cup/30g raw walnuts, or other nut

DRESSING: In a blender or food processor, combine all the ingredients for the dressing and blend well, scraping down the sides as needed, until smooth. If the dressing is too thick for your liking, add up to ⅓ cup/80ml of water and blend to incorporate. Taste to adjust the seasonings. Transfer the dressing to a container with a tight-fitting lid and refrigerate until ready to serve.

SALAD: Preheat the oven to 425°F/220°C/gas mark 7. Arrange the beetroots in a baking dish, cover, and bake until tender, 40 to 60 minutes, depending on the size of the beetroots. Remove from the oven, uncover, and allow to cool. When cool enough to handle, remove the skins from the beetroots, if desired. (They should slip off easily.) Slice, dice, or quarter the beetroots and transfer to a large bowl. Finely chop the kale and add to the bowl. Add the black beans and walnuts. Toss gently to combine. When ready to serve, toss the salad with as much of the dressing as desired.

TIP: The Avocado Goddess Dressing is also great over roasted sweet potatoes and steamed cauliflower.

Daily Dozen Foods

✗ BEANS   ✗ GREENS   ✗ OTHER VEGETABLES   ✗ NUTS AND SEEDS   ✗ HERBS AND SPICES

VINEGAR

Hello. My name is Michael, and I am a vinegar-aholic. Yes. I have an entire bar stocked with vinegars with different flavors to complement different dishes. I put strawberry vinegars on peaches, chocolate vinegar on fresh strawberries, smoky vinegar on savory entrées, peach vinegar on mangoes, and, yes, mango vinegar on peaches. When people think of vinegar, distilled white vinegar may pop into their mind, but that belongs under the sink with other natural cleaners, not the store cupboard. The science on the benefits of vinegars inspired me to explore this surprisingly exotic and far-reaching world, and I'm so glad it did. I try to be a really frugal person, but the three things I splurge on are blazing-fast Internet service, fresh dates every fall and exotic vinegars.

BLACK BEAN GAZPACHO SALAD

MAKES: *4* SERVINGS · DIFFICULTY: *easy*

I knew beans were healthy, but I didn't realize just how healthy until all the amazing microbiome research started coming out. I encourage you to get into the (delicious) habit of eating legumes throughout the day. Before I started pressure-cooking my own, I always kept an open tin of beans in the fridge as a reminder to put them in anything and everything, such as this salad, which, taking its cue from the famous chilled soup, features gazpacho ingredients with black beans and a zesty dressing served over greens.

DRESSING

1 teaspoon white miso paste

2 teaspoons blended peeled lime (see page 3)

1 tablespoon nutritional yeast (or yeast flakes)

¼ teaspoon ground cumin, or to taste

SALAD

1½ cups/95g cooked or 1 15.5-ounce/425g BPA-free tin or Tetra Pak salt-free black beans, drained and rinsed

1 ripe tomato, seeded and finely chopped

1 red or yellow pepper, chopped

1 cup/150g chopped cucumber

¼ cup/25g minced red onion

1 garlic clove, minced

1 teaspoon minced jalapeño pepper

5 cups/375g mixed salad greens

1 small ripe Hass avocado

Healthy Hot Sauce (page 8) (optional)

DRESSING: In a small bowl, combine all the dressing ingredients and stir to blend well. Set aside.

SALAD: In a large bowl, combine the black beans, tomato, pepper, cucumber, onion, garlic and jalapeño.

Pour the dressing over the salad and toss lightly. Cover and set aside for 30 minutes, or refrigerate overnight.

Divide the salad greens among individual salad plates and top with the black bean gazpacho. Halve and pit the avocado and cut it into ½-inch/1cm dice. Top the salads with the avocado and Healthy Hot Sauce (if using). Serve at once.

Daily Dozen Foods

✗ BEANS   ✗ GREENS   ✗ OTHER VEGETABLES   ✗ HERBS AND SPICES

SESAME RED CABBAGE & CARROT SLAW

MAKES: *4* SERVINGS · DIFFICULTY: *easy*

I always keep red cabbage in the fridge. It's cheap, colorful and cruciferocious. And, it seems to keep forever, not that it's ever lasted long enough in my household for us to find out. This vibrant slaw is a nice, much more flavorful change from the typical heavy, mayonnaise-covered coleslaw – and way better for you!

DRESSING

2 tablespoons tahini

2 tablespoons rice vinegar

2 teaspoons blended peeled lemon (see page 3)

2 teaspoons Date Syrup (page 3)

1 teaspoon grated fresh ginger

1 teaspoon white miso paste

SLAW

3 cups/300g shredded red cabbage

1 large carrot, grated

12 mange tout, cut diagonally into thin matchsticks

2 spring onions, minced

1 cup/100g red grapes, halved

2 tablespoons chopped fresh coriander (optional)

2 tablespoons sesame seeds

DRESSING: In a small bowl, combine all of the dressing ingredients with 2 tablespoons of water. Stir well to blend and set aside.

SLAW: In a large bowl, combine the cabbage, carrot, mange tout, spring onions, grapes and coriander (if using). Pour on the dressing and toss gently to coat. Taste and adjust the seasoning as desired. Sprinkle with the sesame seeds. Refrigerate, covered, until ready to serve.

CABBAGE

Antioxidants are your body's defense squad, charged with destroying DNA-damaging free radicals. No need to buy some exotic, so-called superfruit to get them, though. According to a USDA database of common foods, red cabbage provides some of the highest levels of antioxidants per dollar.[110] In fact, red cabbages may have nearly three times the antioxidant power per dollar than do blueberries.[111]

Daily Dozen Foods

✗ OTHER FRUITS ✗ CRUCIFEROUS VEGETABLES ✗ OTHER VEGETABLES ✗ NUTS AND SEEDS ✗ HERBS AND SPICES

CHOPPED VEGETABLE SALAD

MAKES: *4* SERVINGS · DIFFICULTY: *easy*

One of the great things about this recipe is that it's really flexible, so you can cater to whatever you're in the mood for tasting and enjoying. Mix and match ingredients, leaving out any you don't like or may not have on hand and adding other favorites.

1 small head romaine lettuce, chopped into bite-sized pieces

2 radishes, chopped

1 ripe tomato, chopped

1 cup/150g chopped cucumber

½ small orange or red pepper, chopped

½ cup/50g chopped celery

3 artichoke hearts, chopped

1½ cups/90g cooked or 1 15.5-ounce/425g BPA-free tin or Tetra Pak cannellini beans, drained and rinsed

Ranch Dressing (page 7)

In a large bowl, combine the lettuce, radishes, tomato, cucumber, pepper, celery, artichoke hearts and cannellini beans.

Drizzle the Ranch Dressing onto the salad and toss to combine.

DIY SALAD BAR

Keep a selection of salad ingredients prepped so your own personal salad bar is ready whenever you get a craving. Wash and spin-dry salad greens; mix up a few of the dressings in this chapter and keep a variety of washed, sliced and diced veggies in tightly covered containers so all you have to do is create your salad masterpiece. Keep handy store cupboard ingredient add-ins, such as nuts and dried fruit. For variety, change up the greens you use in salads, try different vinegars in the dressings, and add new fruit, veggie and nut combos.

Daily Dozen Foods

✗ BEANS   ✗ GREENS   ✗ OTHER VEGETABLES   ✗ NUTS AND SEEDS   ✗ HERBS AND SPICES

MANGO-AVOCADO-KALE SALAD WITH GINGER-SESAME ORANGE DRESSING

MAKES: *4* SERVINGS · DIFFICULTY: *easy*

Mangoes are one of my favorite fruits. I just love their taste and texture. But I've recently discovered a new fruit I love even more – the papaya, North America's largest native fruit. If you're lucky enough to find a papaya, you can use it in this salad instead of mango.

DRESSING

½ orange, peeled

1 tablespoon rice vinegar

2 tablespoons tahini

1½ teaspoons grated fresh ginger

1 garlic clove, minced

1 tablespoon minced spring onion

2 teaspoons minced fresh parsley or coriander

1 teaspoon white miso paste

1 teaspoon Date Syrup (page 3)

1 ¼-inch/5mm piece fresh turmeric, grated (or ¼ teaspoon ground)

⅛ teaspoon cayenne pepper (optional)

SALAD

5 cups/335g chopped red kale or baby spinach leaves

1 ripe mango, peeled, pitted and cut into ½-inch/1cm dice

1 ripe Hass avocado, peeled, pitted and cut into ½-inch/1cm dice

DRESSING: In a mini-blender or small food processor, combine all the dressing ingredients and blend until smooth. Set aside.

SALAD: In a large bowl, combine the kale, mango and avocado. Pour on as much of the dressing as desired and toss gently to combine.

NOTE: If you don't have a mini-blender or small food processor, you may want to double the dressing recipe to make in a larger machine (and then save half for another day).

Daily Dozen Foods

✗ OTHER FRUITS   ✗ GREENS   ✗ NUTS AND SEEDS   ✗ HERBS AND SPICES

SUPER SALAD WITH GARLIC CAESAR DRESSING & HEMP HEARTS

MAKES: *4* SERVINGS · DIFFICULTY: *easy*

Add bite-sized dices of steamed or sautéed tempeh to this salad for a pretty perfect entrée.

DRESSING

2 garlic cloves, crushed

2 tablespoons nutritional yeast (or yeast flakes)

1 tablespoon almond butter

1 tablespoon blended peeled lemon (see page 3)

1 tablespoon white miso paste

1 tablespoon minced fresh parsley

1 teaspoon salt-free whole-grain mustard

1 ¼-inch/5mm piece fresh turmeric, grated (or ¼ teaspoon ground)

1 teaspoon Savory Spice Blend (page 4), or to taste

SALAD

1 head romaine lettuce, trimmed and torn into small pieces

1 bunch watercress, stemmed and chopped, or 2 cups/550g baby spinach

1 cup/175g halved cherry tomatoes

1 carrot, shredded

3 tablespoons hulled hemp seeds (hemp hearts)

DRESSING: In a blender, combine ½ cup/120ml of water with all the dressing ingredients and blend until smooth. Taste and adjust the seasoning to your liking. Set aside.

SALAD: In a large bowl, combine all the salad ingredients, toss lightly with the dressing, and serve.

Daily Dozen Foods

✗ GREENS   ✗ OTHER VEGETABLES   ✗ NUTS AND SEEDS   ✗ HERBS AND SPICES

PISTACHIO-SPINACH SALAD WITH STRAWBERRY BALSAMIC DRESSING

MAKES: *4* SERVINGS · DIFFICULTY: *easy*

This fancy-looking salad is incredibly easy to make. If fresh strawberries are unavailable, substitute frozen berries that have been thawed to room temperature. (Half our freezer is stocked with frozen berries, and the other half with frozen greens!)

DRESSING

1 cup/200g strawberries, hulled and halved

1 tablespoon chopped shallot

¼ cup/60ml balsamic vinegar

1 tablespoon Date Syrup (page 3)

½ teaspoon salt-free whole-grain mustard

1 teaspoon fresh thyme, or ½ teaspoon dried

½ teaspoon poppy seeds

¼ teaspoon ground black pepper

SALAD

8 cups/1.8kg baby spinach

½ cucumber, halved and thinly sliced

¼ cup/38g raw pistachios

DRESSING: In a blender, combine the strawberries, shallot, vinegar, Date Syrup, mustard and thyme. Blend until smooth. Stir in the poppy seeds and black pepper and set aside.

SALAD: In a large bowl, combine all the salad ingredients, dress to your liking, and toss lightly to coat.

Daily Dozen Foods

X BERRIES   X GREENS   X OTHER VEGETABLES   X NUTS AND SEEDS   X HERBS AND SPICES

BLACK BEAN BURGERS

SLOPPY JACKS

CURRIED CHICKPEA WRAPS

SPINACH & MUSHROOM BLACK BEAN BURRITOS

VERACRUZ TEMPEH LETTUCE WRAPS

BEETROOT BURGERS

BEANS & GREENS QUESADILLAS

BURGERS, WRAPS AND MORE

Beetroot. Black beans. Tempeh. Chickpeas. Teff. Jackfruit.
The recipes in this chapter will introduce you to amazing
flavors bursting from creative takes on traditional dishes.
Say goodbye to artery-clogging burgers!

BLACK BEAN BURGERS

MAKES: *4* SERVINGS · DIFFICULTY: *easy*

There can never be enough ways to get beans into your daily meals. This is one of the best. Serve on toasted 100% whole-grain bread with all the fixings. These burgers freeze well, so consider doubling the recipe so you'll have them ready for just-thaw-and-indulge moments.

1 cup/100g rolled oats

½ cup/55g walnut pieces

1 ¼-inch/5mm piece fresh turmeric, grated (or ¼ teaspoon ground)

½ cup/75g chopped red onion

⅓ cup/35g chopped mushrooms

1½ cups/95g cooked or 1 15-ounce/425g BPA-free tin or Tetra Pak salt-free black beans, well rinsed and drained

2 tablespoons tahini or almond butter

1 tablespoon ground flaxseeds (or linseeds)

1 tablespoon nutritional yeast (or yeast flakes)

1 tablespoon chopped fresh parsley

2 teaspoons white miso paste

1 teaspoon onion powder

½ teaspoon garlic powder

½ teaspoon smoked paprika

1 teaspoon Savory Spice Blend (page 4)

Pulse the oats, walnuts and turmeric in a food processor until they are finely ground. Add the onion, mushrooms, beans, tahini and flaxseeds and pulse until well combined. Add the remaining ingredients and pulse to mix well.

Pinch some of the mixture between your thumb and index finger to test whether it holds together. If the mixture is too wet, add more oats. If the mixture is too dry, add a little water, 1 tablespoon at a time. Transfer the mixture to a work surface and divide into four equal portions. Shape each into a patty about ½-inch/1cm thick and transfer to a plate. Refrigerate for 30 minutes.

Preheat the oven to 375°F/190°C/gas mark 5.

Line a baking sheet with a silicone mat or baking parchment and arrange the burgers on it. Bake until hot and lightly browned, turning once, about 25 minutes. Serve hot, as desired.

Daily Dozen Foods

✗ BEANS ✗ OTHER VEGETABLES ✗ FLAXSEEDS ✗ NUTS AND SEEDS ✗ HERBS AND SPICES ✗ WHOLE GRAINS

SLOPPY JACKS

MAKES: *4* SERVINGS · DIFFICULTY: *easy*

Jackfruit is native to Southern Asia and has been cultivated for as long as six thousand years. Despite its popularity and long culinary history overseas, it's just starting to make a name for itself in the United States because of its versatile texture and interesting flavor – a mix of mango, banana, apple and pineapple. Jackfruit is low in calories and fat, and rich in fiber. You may be able to find fresh jackfruit in Asian markets, or you can just buy it tinned, as I normally do.

1 20-ounce/550g BPA-free tin jackfruit (packed in water, not syrup), drained and rinsed

1 tablespoon nutritional yeast (or yeast flakes)

1 teaspoon Savory Spice Blend (page 4)

½ teaspoon smoked paprika

½ teaspoon chilli powder

1 small red onion, minced

½ red pepper, seeded and minced

¾ cup/170g jarred or Tetra Pak salt-free passata

2 tablespoons date sugar

1 tablespoon salt-free whole-grain mustard

4 slices 100% whole-grain bread

Blot the drained and rinsed jackfruit dry with kitchen paper or a clean tea towel. Remove and discard any hard pieces of its core. Transfer the jackfruit to a bowl and add the nutritional yeast, Savory Spice Blend, paprika and chilli powder. Toss to coat and set aside.

Heat ½ cup/120ml of water in a large frying pan over medium heat. Add the onion and pepper, cover, and cook until soft, about 5 minutes. Stir in the passata, date sugar and mustard. Add the coated jackfruit and reduce the heat to low. Cover and simmer for 25 to 30 minutes, stirring frequently, adding a little more water, 1 tablespoon at a time, if needed so the mixture doesn't stick to the frying pan. As the jackfruit cooks, use two forks to shred it into smaller pieces. Cook uncovered for the final 5 minutes to thicken the sauce. To serve, spoon the jackfruit mixture onto the bread and serve hot.

Daily Dozen Foods

✗ OTHER FRUITS   ✗ OTHER VEGETABLES   ✗ HERBS AND SPICES   ✗ WHOLE GRAINS

CURRIED CHICKPEA WRAPS

MAKES: *4* WRAPS · DIFFICULTY: *easy*

One of the ingredients of curry powder, which is one of my favorite spice mixes, is turmeric. Besides being so good for you, turmeric gives the blend its beautiful yellow color. The curried chickpea filling in this recipe is also great in lettuce wraps or served as a dip. Try it with Three-Seed Crackers (page 34) for a flavorful starter or snack.

1½ cups/255g cooked or 1 15.5-ounce/425g BPA-free tin or Tetra Pak salt-free chickpeas, drained and rinsed

1½ teaspoons curry powder, or to taste

1 teaspoon blended peeled lemon (see page 3)

1 teaspoon date sugar

¼ teaspoon white miso paste

Savory Spice Blend (page 4)

½ cup/50g chopped celery

⅓ cup/17g shredded carrot

⅓ cup/50g chopped cashews

⅓ cup/50g raisins

1 firm sweet apple, cored and chopped

1 tablespoon chopped spring onion

4 100% whole-grain tortillas

2 cups/150g shredded lettuce

In a food processor, combine 1 cup/170g of the chickpeas with the curry powder, lemon, date sugar, miso and Savory Spice Blend to taste with 3 to 4 tablespoons of water. Process until smooth. Add the remaining ½ cup/85g of chickpeas and the celery, carrot, cashews, raisins, apple and spring onion, and pulse just to combine and break up the chickpeas a bit. Taste and adjust the seasonings, if needed.

To assemble, divide the chickpea mixture evenly onto the tortillas and top each with the lettuce. Tightly roll up each of the tortillas to make a wrap. Cut each wrap in half and serve immediately.

CHICKPEAS

The more chickpeas (and other legumes) you eat, the healthier you are. In one study, researchers divided overweight subjects into two groups. The first group was asked to eat 1kg a week of chickpeas, lentils, split peas or haricot beans – but not to change their diet in any other way. The second group was asked to simply cut out 500 calories a day from their diet.

Guess who got healthier? The group directed to eat *more* food. Eating chickpeas and other beans was shown to be just as effective at slimming waistlines and improving blood sugar control as it is at cutting calories. The legume group also gained additional benefits in the form of improved cholesterol and insulin regulation.[112]

Daily Dozen Foods

✗ BEANS ✗ OTHER FRUITS ✗ GREENS ✗ OTHER VEGETABLES ✗ NUTS AND SEEDS ✗ HERBS AND SPICES ✗ WHOLE GRAINS

SPINACH & MUSHROOM BLACK BEAN BURRITOS

MAKES: *4* SERVINGS · DIFFICULTY: *easy*

Spinach is not my favorite green. I love all dark green leafies, but I'm more likely to go for a cruciferous one, such as kale or rocket. Spinach is a great option for newbies, though. It doesn't have a strong distinctive flavor, so you can blend handfuls into a smoothie and hardly taste it. Spinach also fits well into foods like burritos, such as this nutritious one featuring mushrooms and black beans. This filling is so good you shouldn't save it only for burritos. Make a double batch so you have it on hand to heat and eat whenever and however you want.

1½ cups/95g cooked or 1 15.5-ounce/425g BPA-free tin or Tetra Pak salt-free black beans, drained and rinsed

½ cup/75g minced red onion

2 garlic cloves, minced

2 cups/200g chopped mushrooms

4 cups/900g baby spinach

1 tablespoon nutritional yeast (or yeast flakes)

Savory Spice Blend (page 4)

Cayenne pepper

Healthy Hot Sauce (page 8)

4 100% whole-grain tortillas

Summer Salsa (page 41)

In a bowl, mash the black beans with a fork or potato ricer and set aside.

Heat ¼ cup/60ml of water in a frying pan and add the onion and garlic. Cook, stirring occasionally, until softened, about 5 minutes. Stir in the mushrooms and cook for 3 minutes longer to soften. Add the spinach and cook, stirring, until the spinach is wilted. Add the mashed black beans and continue to cook, stirring, until the liquid is absorbed. Stir in the nutritional yeast, Savory Spice Blend, cayenne and hot sauce to taste. Taste and adjust the seasonings to your liking.

To serve, spoon a quarter of the filling down the center of each tortilla. Add more hot sauce, if desired, and roll up each burrito, tucking in the sides as you do so. Serve immediately or, one at a time, place each filled burrito in a hot non-stick frying pan for a minute or two – just long enough to lightly brown the outside of the tortillas. Serve with the Summer Salsa.

Daily Dozen Foods

X BEANS   X GREENS   X OTHER VEGETABLES   X HERBS AND SPICES   X WHOLE GRAINS

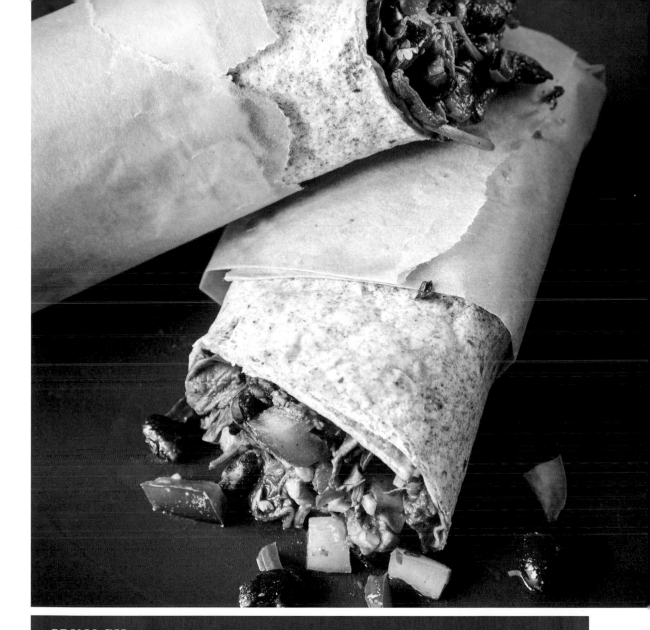

SPINACH

Popeye was right when he bragged he was strong to the finish because he ate his spinach. Of all the food groups analyzed by a team of Harvard University researchers, greens turned out to be associated with the strongest protection against major chronic diseases,[113] including up to about a 20 percent reduction in risk for both heart attacks[114] and strokes[115] associated with every additional daily serving. Comparing spinach, round lettuce, endive, radicchio and romaine lettuce, Cornell University researchers found that spinach was best at suppressing the growth of breast cancer, brain tumor, kidney cancer, lung cancer, pediatric brain tumor, pancreatic cancer, prostate cancer and stomach cancer cells in vitro.[116]

VERACRUZ TEMPEH LETTUCE WRAPS

MAKES: *4* SERVINGS (2 WRAPS PER SERVING) · DIFFICULTY: *moderate*

Nori flakes help give these crunchy wraps a taste of the sea. Look for nori and other sea vegetables in natural food stores, Asian shops or online.

8 ounces/225g tempeh, cut into ¼-inch/5mm dice

2 teaspoons chilli powder

2 teaspoons ground cumin

½ teaspoon cayenne pepper

1 small red onion, chopped

2 garlic cloves, minced

1 or 2 jalapeño peppers, seeded and minced

3 Roma tomatoes, chopped

1 teaspoon nori or dulse flakes

1 tablespoon blended peeled lime (see page 3)

8 large romaine or round lettuce leaves, for wraps

1 ripe Hass avocado, peeled, pitted and chopped

½ cup/25g chopped fresh coriander (optional)

Healthy Hot Sauce (page 8) or Summer Salsa (page 41) (optional)

Steam the tempeh in a steamer basket over boiling water for 15 minutes and then set aside, uncovered.

In a shallow bowl, combine the chilli powder, cumin and cayenne; then add the steamed tempeh, tossing lightly to coat.

Heat ¼ cup/60ml of water in a frying pan over medium-high heat. Add the onion, garlic and jalapeño and cook for 5 minutes or until soft, adding a little more water if needed so the ingredients don't burn. Stir in the tomatoes and nori and cook until most of the liquid evaporates, about 3 minutes longer. Add the seasoned tempeh and lime and continue to cook until lightly browned, about 4 minutes.

To assemble, spoon some of the filling onto a lettuce leaf and top with some avocado, coriander (if using) and Healthy Hot Sauce or Summer Salsa to taste (if using). Repeat with the remaining ingredients and serve.

Daily Dozen Foods

✗ BEANS   ✗ OTHER FRUITS   ✗ GREENS   ✗ OTHER VEGETABLES   ✗ HERBS AND SPICES

BEETROOT BURGERS

MAKES: *6* BURGERS · DIFFICULTY: *moderate*

What's teff? An Ethiopian grain, teff may have been cultivated as many as six thousand years ago. It is tiny – 150 grains of teff equal the weight of just a single grain of wheat. The word comes from an Ethiopian root that means 'lost', because if you drop a grain of it, you are not likely to find it again. As such, teff cooks more quickly than other grains.

½ cup/75g minced red onion

2 garlic cloves, minced

1 cup/150g finely grated raw beetroot

1 cup/100g minced mushrooms

½ teaspoon smoked paprika

½ teaspoon mustard powder

½ teaspoon ground cumin

½ teaspoon ground coriander

1 ¼-inch/5mm piece fresh turmeric, grated (or ¼ teaspoon ground)

1 ½ cups/95g cooked or 1 15-ounce/425g BPA-free tin or Tetra Pak salt-free black beans, rinsed and well drained

1 cup/250g cooked brown, red or black rice; teff; or quinoa; well drained and blotted dry

1 tablespoon ground flaxseeds (or linseeds)

1 tablespoon white miso paste

½ cup/50g rolled oats, ground into coarse flour

½ cup/55g ground walnuts

6 100% whole-grain buns

Heat ¼ cup/60ml of water in a large frying pan over medium heat. Add the onion and cook until softened, about 5 minutes. Stir in the garlic and then add the beetroot and mushrooms. Sprinkle on the paprika, mustard, cumin, coriander and turmeric. Cook until the vegetables are softened and the liquid is absorbed, about 4 minutes.

In a large bowl, mash the beans well to break them up. Add the cooked grain, flaxseeds and miso. Mash the mixture to combine and then add the oats and walnuts, then the cooked vegetables. Combine until the mixture holds together when pressed between your thumb and forefinger. Divide the mixture into six equal portions and use your hands to shape them into balls. Press the balls into patties and transfer them to a plate. Refrigerate for a minimum of 30 minutes.

Preheat the oven to 375°F/190°C/gas mark 5. Line a baking sheet with a silicone mat or baking parchment and arrange the burgers on it. Bake for 30 minutes, gently flipping the patties about halfway through. Serve hot with or without a bun and your favorite condiments.

NOTE: Be careful when grating beetroots – their bright red color can stain!

SOYA

Soya bean consumption helps reduce menopausal hot-flash symptoms,[117] as well as decrease a woman's risk of breast cancer.[118] In fact, women diagnosed with breast cancer who ate more soya lived significantly longer and had a significantly lower risk of breast cancer recurrence than those who ate less.[119]

Daily Dozen Foods

✗ BEANS   ✗ OTHER VEGETABLES   ✗ NUTS AND SEEDS   ✗ HERBS AND SPICES   ✗ WHOLE GRAINS

BEANS & GREENS QUESADILLAS

MAKES: *4* SERVINGS · DIFFICULTY: *easy*

Who needs queso when you can enjoy quesadillas filled with a zesty blend of beans and greens?

1 small red onion, minced

3 garlic cloves, minced

1 bunch (about 5 cups/1.1kg) chard or red kale, finely chopped

2 Roma tomatoes, chopped

1½ cups/95g cooked or 1 15.5-ounce/425g BPA-free tin or Tetra Pak salt-free cannellini beans, drained and rinsed

2 tablespoons nutritional yeast (or yeast flakes)

1 teaspoon chilli powder

Savory Spice Blend (page 4) (optional)

Healthy Hot Sauce (page 8) (optional)

4 (10-inch/25cm) 100% whole-grain tortillas

Summer Salsa (page 41) (optional)

Heat ¼ cup/60ml of water in a pan over medium heat. Add the onion and garlic and cook until softened, about 5 minutes. Add the chard and tomatoes, and continue to cook, stirring, until the greens are tender and the liquid is cooked off, about 5 minutes longer.

While the greens are cooking, mash the beans in a bowl and stir in the nutritional yeast, chilli powder and Savory Spice Blend and Healthy Hot Sauce to taste (if using). Mix well.

Drain off any remaining liquid from the greens mixture and then stir into the bean mixture. Taste and adjust the seasonings, if needed.

Divide the filling among the tortillas, spreading it evenly over the bottom half of each. Fold the top half of the tortilla over the filling, pressing down lightly to hold the halves together. Place two of the quesadillas in a large nonstick frying pan or griddle over medium heat. Cook until lightly browned on both sides, turning once, about 3 minutes per side. Repeat with the remaining quesadillas. To serve, cut each quesadilla into three or four wedges and arrange on plates. Serve with Summer Salsa, if desired.

Daily Dozen Foods

✗ BEANS ✗ GREENS ✗ OTHER VEGETABLES ✗ HERBS AND SPICES ✗ WHOLE GRAINS

VERY VEGGIE MAINS

Thankfully, the days of relegating vegetables to the side
of our plates are fading fast and with good reason.
Bite for bite, you just can't beat veggies. The dishes in
this chapter are innovative, delicious and the perfect
way to spotlight vegetables on center stage!

COURGETTE NOODLES WITH
AVOCADO-CASHEW ALFREDO

PESTO CARROT NOODLES WITH
WHITE BEANS & TOMATOES

SPAGHETTI SQUASH ARRABIATA

ROASTED VEGETABLE LASAGNA

STUFFED PORTOBELLOS WITH
HERBED MUSHROOM GRAVY

WHOLE ROASTED CAULIFLOWER
WITH LEMON TAHINI SAUCE

VEGETABLE STACKS WITH
TOMATO-RED PEPPER COULIS

CAULIFLOWER STEAKS
WITH CHERMOULA SAUCE

PORTOBELLOS & GREENS ON TOAST

COURGETTE NOODLES WITH AVOCADO-CASHEW ALFREDO

MAKES: *4* SERVINGS · DIFFICULTY: *moderate*

If you don't have a spiralizer, don't worry. You can still make courgette noodles right at home. Simply use an everyday vegetable peeler to scrape long, thin strands from the courgettes.

---

1 cup/150g raw cashews, soaked for 4 hours and then drained

2 tablespoons nutritional yeast (or yeast flakes)

2 teaspoons white miso paste

1½ cups/360ml Vegetable Broth (page 6) or water

½ ripe Hass avocado, peeled and pitted

1 tablespoon blended peeled lemon (see page 3)

4 to 6 medium courgettes, trimmed and spiralized or cut into long, thin, noodle-like strips

1 cup/175g cherry tomatoes, halved lengthwise

Ground black pepper or chilli flakes

2 tablespoons minced fresh parsley or basil

Nutty Parm (page 4), to serve

Grind the drained cashews in a high-speed blender. Add the nutritional yeast, miso and broth and blend until smooth. Add the avocado and lemon and blend until smooth, adding more broth, 1 tablespoon at a time, if the sauce is too thick. Set aside.

Steam the courgette noodles over boiling water until tender, 2 to 4 minutes. Set aside.

In a large saucepan or deep frying pan, warm the cashew sauce over low heat, stirring often. Add the courgette noodles and tomatoes. Stir gently until the vegetables are heated through, about 5 minutes. If the sauce is too thick, add a little more broth to reach your desired consistency. When hot, serve at once, sprinkled with black pepper to taste, the parsley and Nutty Parm.

SPIRALIZING

Traditional noodles are made of grains, but thanks to the spiralizer, you can make your own noodles out of vegetables. The spiralizer is an inexpensive tool that lets you turn fresh veggies into veggie-noodles.

Daily Dozen Foods

✗ OTHER FRUITS   ✗ OTHER VEGETABLES   ✗ NUTS AND SEEDS   ✗ HERBS AND SPICES

PESTO CARROT NOODLES WITH WHITE BEANS & TOMATOES

MAKES: *4* SERVINGS · DIFFICULTY: *moderate*

Pesto is like a magic act: You take a green leafy vegetable (basil) and with just a little work, pesto presto! You turn it into a delicious sauce! The pesto in this recipe can also be enjoyed with your favorite whole-grain or bean pasta.

3 garlic cloves

1 teaspoon white miso paste

3 cups/90g basil leaves

⅓ cup/40g almonds or walnuts

2 tablespoons nutritional yeast (or yeast flakes)

½ cup/120ml Vegetable Broth (page 6) or water

Ground black pepper

4 large carrots

1½ cups/95g cooked or 1 15.5-ounce/425g BPA-free tin or Tetra Pak salt-free cannellini beans, drained and rinsed

1 cup/175g cherry tomatoes, halved lengthwise

Nutty Parm (page 4), to serve

In a food processor, combine the garlic and miso and process until the garlic is minced. Add the basil, nuts and nutritional yeast and process until finely minced. Add the broth and black pepper to taste, and process until smooth, adding a little more broth if needed to achieve the desired texture for your pesto sauce. Set aside.

Cut the carrots into long, thin strips, using a spiralizer, mandoline or vegetable peeler. Steam the carrot noodles until tender, 5 to 7 minutes. In a shallow bowl, combine the carrot noodles with the beans, tomatoes and pesto sauce and toss gently to combine. Sprinkle with Nutty Parm and serve.

WALNUTS

Walnuts are probably the healthiest nuts, containing the most omega-3s and antioxidant power. They are my nuts of choice, and I often swap out other nuts in recipes for these to maximize the nutritional value of my meals.

Daily Dozen Foods

X BEANS   X OTHER VEGETABLES   X NUTS AND SEEDS   X HERBS AND SPICES

SPAGHETTI SQUASH ARRABIATA

MAKES: *4* SERVINGS · DIFFICULTY: *easy*

Remember, as with most vegetables, the more colorful the squash, the more likely it's packed with antioxidants.

1 large (3-pound/1.3kg) spaghetti squash, cut in half

3 garlic cloves, minced

3 cups/675g fresh, jarred or Tetra Pak tomatoes, finely diced

2 tablespoons jarred tomato purée

1 teaspoon balsamic vinegar

1 teaspoon white miso paste

1 teaspoon dried basil

½ teaspoon chilli flakes, or to taste

Savory Spice Blend (page 4)

¼ cup/4 tablespoons minced fresh parsley

Ground black pepper

Nutty Parm (page 4)

Preheat the oven to 350°F/180°C/gas mark 4. Place the squash halves in a large baking dish, cut side up. Add 1 to 2 inches/2.5 to 5cm of water and tightly cover the dish. Bake until tender, 45 to 60 minutes.

While the squash is baking, make the sauce in a large frying pan: Heat 2 tablespoons of water over medium heat. Add the garlic and cook for 1 minute to soften. Stir in all the remaining ingredients, except the Nutty Parm, and cook for 5 minutes longer. Keep warm.

When the squash is done baking, remove and discard its seeds. Use a fork to scrape the squash in strands and place in a large bowl. Add the sauce and toss gently to combine. Sprinkle with Nutty Parm and serve.

TIP: This arrabiata sauce also tastes great tossed with courgette noodles or whole-grain pasta.

NUTS IN THE RAW

It's healthiest to eat nuts raw. When high-fat and high-protein foods are exposed to temperatures above 250°F/120°C, advanced glycation end products, or AGEs, are created. Appropriately acronymed, these so-called glycotoxins are thought to accelerate the aging process. The highest levels are found in grilled, roasted, fried and barbecued meat, but AGEs can also occur when plant foods high in fat and protein, such as soya foods or nuts, are grilled or toasted.

Daily Dozen Foods

✗ OTHER VEGETABLES   ✗ NUTS AND SEEDS   ✗ HERBS AND SPICES

ROASTED VEGETABLE LASAGNA

MAKES: *6* SERVINGS · DIFFICULTY: *moderate*

One of the wonderful things about lasagna is being able to truly make it your own. Not crazy about aubergine? Use sliced portobello mushrooms instead (as I do). Want to bulk it up? Add some crumbled steamed tempeh to the tomato sauce. And, as always, consider adding chopped greens to this – and everything else!

1 head cauliflower, cut vertically into ¼-inch/5mm slices

1 courgette, cut into ⅛-inch/3mm slices

1 aubergine, cut into ⅛-inch/3mm slices

1 red pepper, seeded and chopped

12 100% whole-grain lasagna sheets

1½ cups/95g cooked or 1 15.5-ounce/425g BPA-free tin or Tetra Pak cannellini beans, drained, rinsed and mashed

¼ cup/15g nutritional yeast (or yeast flakes)

¼ cup/4 tablespoons minced fresh parsley

½ cup/120ml Almond Milk (page 2)

1 teaspoon blended peeled lemon (see page 3)

1 teaspoon white miso paste

1 teaspoon dried oregano

1 teaspoon dried basil

1 teaspoon garlic powder

1 teaspoon onion powder

¼ teaspoon chilli flakes, or to taste

¼ teaspoon ground black pepper

3 cups/675g jarred or homemade marinara sauce

¼ cup/25g Nutty Parm (page 4)

Daily Dozen Foods

Preheat the oven to 425°F/220°C/gas mark 7. Line two large baking sheets with silicone mats or baking parchment. Arrange the cauliflower on one of the prepared baking sheets and the courgette and aubergine on the other. Sprinkle the chopped pepper over the courgette and aubergine. Place both pans of vegetables in the oven and roast until the veggies are tender, about 20 minutes, turning once about halfway through.

While the vegetables are roasting, cook the lasagna sheets according to the packet instructions. Drain and set aside.

Remove the roasted vegetables from the oven and set aside to cool. Lower the oven temperature to 350°F/180°C/gas mark 4.

Transfer the roasted cauliflower to a food processor and pulse until it is finely chopped. Place the cauliflower in a large bowl and add the remaining ingredients, except the marinara sauce and Nutty Parm. Mix well.

To assemble, spread a layer of marinara sauce on the bottom of a 9 × 13-inch/23 x 32cm baking dish. Top the sauce with a layer of lasagna. Cover the lasagna sheets with half of the roasted vegetables, topped with half of the cauliflower mixture. Add another layer of lasagna, topped with more sauce. Once again cover the lasagna with roasted vegetables, and then the cauliflower mixture. Repeat this layering process, ending with a layer of lasagna sheets topped with sauce. Sprinkle Nutty Parm on top. Cover and bake for 30 to 40 minutes, or until hot and bubbling. Remove from the oven and let stand for 10 minutes before cutting and serving.

X BEANS   X OTHER VEGETABLES   X NUTS AND SEEDS   X HERBS AND SPICES   X WHOLE GRAINS

STUFFED PORTOBELLOS WITH HERBED MUSHROOM GRAVY

MAKES: *4* SERVINGS · DIFFICULTY: *easy*

If I had been preparing a Daily *Baker's* Dozen, mushrooms would probably have made my list. Though the evidence isn't quite as strong, there's a lot of interesting new research that touts the benefits mushrooms offer, especially on improving immune function. If I don't have fresh mushrooms on hand, then dried will do. I cook them in soups, add them to pasta sauces or make them the star player, as in this dish.

4 large portobello mushroom caps, stems removed

2 spring onions, coarsely chopped

2 garlic cloves, minced

3 cups/675g spinach leaves, loosely packed

1½ cups/260g cooked or 1 15.5-ounce/425g BPA-free tin or Tetra Pak salt-free chickpeas, drained and rinsed

2 tablespoons tahini

2 tablespoons nutritional yeast (or yeast flakes)

2 tablespoons white miso paste

1 teaspoon blended peeled lemon (see page 3)

½ teaspoon onion powder

½ teaspoon smoked paprika

Ground black pepper

½ cup/25g 100% whole-grain bread crumbs

2 tablespoons ground flaxseeds (or linseeds)

2 shallots, finely minced

2 cups/200g chopped, assorted fresh mushrooms

1½ cups/360ml Vegetable Broth (page 6)

1 teaspoon dried thyme

½ teaspoon dried sage

2 tablespoons chopped fresh parsley

Preheat the oven to 400°F/200°C/gas mark 6. Arrange the mushroom caps, stem side down, in a large baking dish with ¼ cup/60ml of water and bake for 10 minutes to soften.

While the mushrooms are baking, make the stuffing: In a food processor, combine the spring onions, garlic, spinach and chickpeas and process until finely minced. Add the tahini, nutritional yeast, 1 tablespoon of the miso, and the lemon, onion powder, paprika and black pepper to taste. Pulse to combine. Add the bread crumbs and flaxseeds and pulse once again to combine while retaining some texture in the chickpeas. Flip over the baked mushrooms and spoon the stuffing mixture into the mushroom caps, gently pressing the stuffing into each cap. Bake for about 20 minutes, or until the mushrooms are tender and the stuffing is hot.

While the stuffed mushrooms are baking, make the gravy: Heat 2 tablespoons of water in a frying pan over medium heat. Add the shallot and cook until soft, about 3 minutes. Add the chopped, assorted mushrooms and cook for 2 to 3 minutes to soften. Stir in the broth, remaining tablespoon of miso, thyme, sage and black pepper to taste. Bring to a boil, then reduce the heat to low and simmer for 5 minutes. Transfer the mixture to a blender or food processor and blend until smooth.

Serve the stuffed mushrooms hot with the gravy spooned over the top and sprinkled with parsley.

TIP: The gravy is also delicious as a topping for the Black Bean Burgers (page 88) and the Red Quinoa Loaf (page 156).

Daily Dozen Foods

✗ BEANS ✗ GREENS ✗ OTHER VEGETABLES ✗ FLAXSEEDS ✗ NUTS AND SEEDS ✗ HERBS AND SPICES

WHOLE ROASTED CAULIFLOWER WITH LEMON TAHINI SAUCE

MAKES: *4* SERVINGS · DIFFICULTY: *easy*

Cauliflower is another nutritious plant that can be served many ways – roasted, boiled, sautéed, grilled, steamed or raw. The whole cauliflower in this dish makes a great-looking centerpiece on the dinner table.

3 garlic cloves, crushed

2 teaspoons white miso paste

1 tablespoon tahini

1½ tablespoons blended peeled lemon (see page 3)

2 tablespoons nutritional yeast (or yeast flakes)

½ teaspoon salt-free whole-grain mustard

1 ¼-inch/5mm piece fresh turmeric, grated (or ¼ teaspoon ground)

Savory Spice Blend (page 4)

1 head cauliflower, leaves and tough stem removed

3 tablespoons chopped fresh parsley

Ground black pepper

In a food processor or blender, combine the garlic and miso and process until the garlic is finely minced. Add ½ cup/120ml of water and the tahini, lemon, nutritional yeast, mustard, turmeric and Savory Spice Blend to taste and blend the sauce until smooth. Set aside.

Bring water to boil in a pan large enough for the cauliflower to be immersed fully. Place the cauliflower carefully in the boiling water. Cover and cook until blanched, about 8 minutes.

Preheat the oven to 400°F/200°C/gas mark 6.

Transfer the cauliflower to a shallow baking dish, stem side down, and add ½ inch/1cm of water. Spoon about half of the sauce on top of the cauliflower and use your fingers to rub the sauce onto the cauliflower. Roast until the cauliflower is tender, about 40 minutes. Stir the parsley and black pepper to taste into the remaining sauce and adjust the seasonings, if needed. Heat the remaining sauce in a small saucepan or microwave. When the cauliflower is ready, transfer it to a platter and top with the remaining sauce. Serve hot.

CAULIFLOWER

If you added only one thing to your diet, consider cruciferous vegetables, such as cauliflower. Less than a single serving a day of cauliflower, broccoli, Brussels sprouts, cabbage or kale may cut the risk of certain cancers progressing by more than half.[120]

Daily Dozen Foods

X CRUCIFEROUS VEGETABLES   X NUTS AND SEEDS   X HERBS AND SPICES

VEGETABLE STACKS WITH TOMATO-RED PEPPER COULIS

MAKES: *4* SERVINGS · DIFFICULTY: *moderate*

This dish takes a little extra time to assemble, but the bit of effort is so very worth it. It's actually a quite simple dish to make and looks very fancy when plated. Perfect for when you want to impress your dining companion!

1 large aubergine, trimmed and cut into 4 round slices about ½ inch/1cm thick

1 large red onion, cut into 4 slices about ½ inch/1cm thick

1 large orange or yellow pepper, sides cut vertically to make 4 square pieces

4 large portobello mushroom caps, gills removed

1 or 2 large ripe tomatoes, cut into 4 slices about ½ inch/1cm thick

3 tablespoons minced red onion

2 plum tomatoes, chopped

2 roasted red peppers (see page 9, or shop-bought)

1 teaspoon white miso paste

1 teaspoon dried basil

½ teaspoon dried thyme

1 ¼-inch/5mm piece fresh turmeric, grated (or ¼ teaspoon ground)

Ground black pepper

Fresh parsley for garnish

Preheat the oven to 425°F/220°C/gas mark 7.

Line two large baking sheets with silicone mats or baking parchment. Arrange the aubergine slices in a single layer on one of the prepared baking sheets. Bake the aubergine until soft, turning once, about 15 minutes. Remove the baking sheet from the oven and set aside to cool; then remove the aubergine from the sheet. Meanwhile, on the second prepared baking sheet, arrange the onion slices in a single layer and bake for 7 to 8 minutes. Turn over the onion slices, place the pepper pieces on the same baking sheet as the onion, and roast until the vegetables are tender, about 15 minutes longer. Set aside to cool. Arrange the mushroom caps, gill side up, on the baking sheet from which the aubergine has been removed. Roast until softened, about 10 minutes. Set aside to cool for a few minutes.

Lower the oven temperature to 350°F/180°C/gas mark 4. Assemble the roasted vegetables in stacks: To begin, leave the four mushroom caps, gill side up, on their baking sheet. Top each cap with a slice of aubergine, followed by a slice of onion, then a pepper slice, topped with a slice of tomato. Cover the baking sheet and bake until the vegetables are hot, about 20 minutes.

While the vegetables are cooking, make the sauce: In a frying pan, heat 3 tablespoons of water over medium heat and add the minced onion. Cover and cook for 4 minutes, or until soft. Stir in the plum tomatoes, roasted peppers, miso, basil, thyme, turmeric and black pepper to taste. Cover and cook until the vegetables are very soft, about 5 minutes longer. Transfer to a food processor and purée the sauce until smooth. Keep warm over low heat until ready to use.

Daily Dozen Foods

𝘟 OTHER VEGETABLES   𝘟 HERBS AND SPICES

When the stacks are ready, use a metal spatula to carefully remove them from the baking dish. Place one stack in the center of each of four dinner plates. Top and surround each stack with the sauce and parsley garnish, and serve hot.

TIP: For a more attractive dish, cut the stackable vegetables slices so they are approximately the same size. Reserve the remaining pieces of the vegetables for another use.

CAULIFLOWER STEAKS WITH CHERMOULA SAUCE

MAKES: *4* SERVINGS · DIFFICULTY: *easy*

Chermoula is a sauce found in Northern African cuisine, most often made of a mixture of herbs, oil, lemon juice, pickled lemons, garlic, cumin and salt. It may also include onion, coriander, ground chilli peppers, black pepper or saffron. It's one of the most dramatic flavors I've tasted and elevates this meaty steak to another level. Serve this dish over quinoa or brown, red or black rice for a spectacular meal.

1 head cauliflower, trimmed, cored and cut into ½-inch/1cm-thick slices

3 garlic cloves, crushed

¾ cup/22g coarsely chopped fresh parsley

¾ cup/38g coarsely chopped fresh coriander

1 ¼-inch/5mm piece fresh turmeric, grated (or ¼ teaspoon ground)

1 teaspoon white miso paste

½ teaspoon ground coriander

½ teaspoon ground cumin

½ teaspoon smoked paprika

¼ teaspoon ground ginger

¼ teaspoon cayenne pepper

1 tablespoon blended peeled lemon (see page 3)

Preheat the oven to 425°F/220°C/gas mark 7.

Arrange the cauliflower slices on a large baking sheet lined with a silicone mat or baking parchment. Roast until just tender, about 15 minutes, turning once halfway through.

In a food processor, combine the garlic, parsley, coriander and turmeric and process until finely minced. Add the miso, coriander, cumin, paprika, ginger, cayenne, lemon and ¼ cup/60ml of water. Process until the sauce is smooth. Set aside.

Remove the roasted cauliflower from the oven and use a metal spatula to transfer it to a shallow serving platter. Serve hot, topped with the sauce.

Daily Dozen Foods

✗ CRUCIFEROUS VEGETABLES   ✗ HERBS AND SPICES

PORTOBELLOS & GREENS ON TOAST

MAKES: *4* SERVINGS · DIFFICULTY: *easy*

As much as I love mushrooms, they are seldom a main dish for me. Portobellos are the exception because they're so hearty and satisfying. This open-faced, knife-and-fork sandwich makes a quick and easy lunch or dinner entrée.

8 to 12 ounces/225 to 350g portobello mushroom caps, thinly sliced

3 spring onions, minced

6 cups/1.3kg chopped spinach or chard

1 teaspoon dried thyme

½ teaspoon smoked paprika

¼ teaspoon ground black pepper

2 tablespoons Umami Sauce (page 5)

½ teaspoon salt-free whole-grain mustard

⅓ cup/80ml Almond Milk (page 2)

4 slices 100% whole-grain bread

2 tablespoons chopped fresh parsley

Heat 2 tablespoons of water in a large frying pan over medium-high heat. Add the portobellos and stir-fry until softened. Add the spring onions and spinach and cook, stirring, for 1 to 2 minutes to wilt the greens. Add the thyme, paprika, black pepper, Umami Sauce, mustard and Almond Milk, stirring to blend well, and cook for 1 to 2 minutes longer to thicken slightly. Keep warm while you toast the bread. Once the bread is toasted, cut the slices in half and arrange them on plates. Top with the portobellos and greens and sprinkle with parsley. Serve warm.

VARIATIONS: Add 1 cup/62g of cooked beans. Serve over brown, black or red rice or another whole grain instead of toast. If you prefer, try shiitakes instead of portobellos. Likewise, you can use kale or tatsoi instead of spinach or chard.

MUSHROOMS

Mushrooms may be able to boost immune function. An Australian study found that people eating a cup of cooked white button mushrooms every day can elevate their saliva IgA levels – antibodies that neutralize and prevent viruses from penetrating into the body – by as much as 50 percent.[123] This appears to translate into fewer viral infections.[124]

Daily Dozen Foods

✗ GREENS   ✗ OTHER VEGETABLES   ✗ HERBS AND SPICES   ✗ WHOLE GRAINS

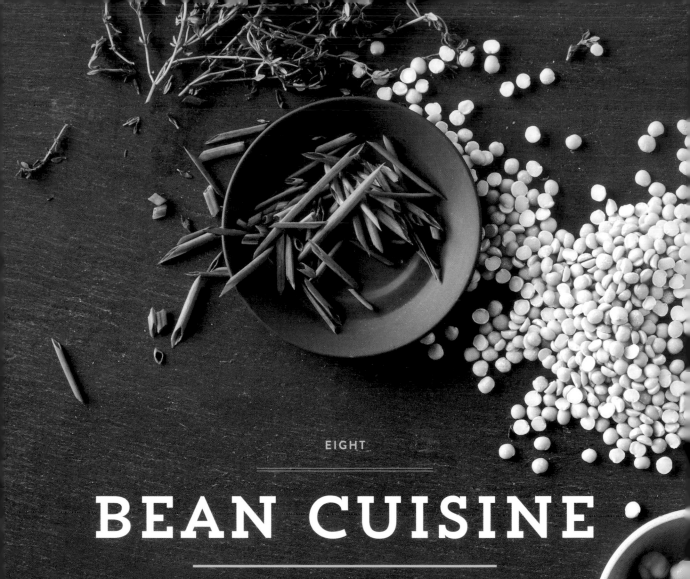

BEAN CUISINE

This chapter features beans every which way, from the more exotic Chickpea & Vegetable Tagine, Bean Patties with Harissa, and Yellow Split Pea Dal with Watercress to Daily Dozen-inspired takes on down-home favorites, such as Smoky Black-Eyed Peas & Spring Greens and Lentil Shepherd's Pie. Recipes using tempeh and Soy Curls are also featured, and I hope you love the Braised Tempeh & Bok Choy with Spicy Ginger Sauce and Louisiana-Style Soy Curls as much as I do.

CHICKPEA & VEGETABLE TAGINE

SMOKY BLACK-EYED PEAS & SPRING GREENS

BRAISED TEMPEH & BOK CHOY
WITH SPICY GINGER SAUCE

CHICKPEA & CAULIFLOWER CURRY

LENTIL SHEPHERD'S PIE

YELLOW SPLIT PEA DAL WITH WATERCRESS

LOUISIANA-STYLE SOY CURLS

BEAN PATTIES WITH HARISSA

CHICKPEA & VEGETABLE TAGINE

MAKES: *4* SERVINGS • DIFFICULTY: *easy*

Lots of spices combine with lots of veggies for a great-tasting dish that is especially good served over quinoa or brown, red or black rice. Common to North African cuisine, *tagine* refers both to the earthenware pot in which the food is cooked as well as the food itself.

1 red onion, chopped

1 carrot, chopped

1 green pepper, seeded and chopped

1 garlic clove, minced

1½ teaspoons minced fresh ginger

2 tablespoons jarred tomato purée

¼ teaspoon ground cinnamon

½ teaspoon ground cumin

½ teaspoon smoked paprika

1 ¼-inch/5mm piece fresh turmeric, grated (or ¼ teaspoon ground)

⅛ to ¼ teaspoon cayenne pepper, or to taste

2 cups/500ml Vegetable Broth (page 6)

1 cup/150g green beans, cut into 1-inch/2.5cm pieces

2 cups/200g diced mushrooms

1½ cups/255g cooked or 1 15.5-ounce/425g BPA free tin or Tetra Pak salt-free chickpeas, drained and rinsed

2 tablespoons minced fresh coriander or parsley

2 teaspoons blended peeled lemon (see page 3)

1 tablespoon raisins or minced dried apricot

Heat ¼ cup/60ml of water in a large saucepan over medium heat. Add the onion, carrot and pepper. Cover and cook for 5 minutes. Stir in the garlic, ginger, tomato purée, cinnamon, cumin, paprika, turmeric and cayenne. Add the broth, green beans, mushrooms and chickpeas and bring to a boil. Reduce the heat to low, cover, and simmer until the vegetables are tender, about 20 minutes. Stir in the coriander, lemon and raisins and cook 5 minutes longer. Taste to adjust the seasonings, and serve hot.

Daily Dozen Foods

✗ BEANS   ✗ OTHER FRUITS   ✗ OTHER VEGETABLES   ✗ HERBS AND SPICES

SMOKY BLACK-EYED PEAS & SPRING GREENS

MAKES: *4* SERVINGS · DIFFICULTY: *easy*

This Southern classic is a delicious way to enjoy your greens. If fresh greens are unavailable, substitute frozen greens or another dark green leafy vegetable, such as kale. I can't get enough of this dish, especially when it's over quinoa or brown, black or red rice.

1½ pounds/675g fresh spring greens, well washed, tough stems removed

1 small red onion, chopped

1 garlic clove, minced

1 teaspoon smoked paprika

1 ¼-inch/5mm piece fresh turmeric, grated (or ¼ teaspoon ground)

Savory Spice Blend (page 4)

1 teaspoon white miso paste

1 14.5-ounce/400g BPA-free tin or Tetra Pak salt-free diced tomatoes, drained

1½ cups/95g cooked or 1 15.5-ounce/425g BPA-free tin or Tetra Pak salt-free black-eyed peas, drained and rinsed

Healthy Hot Sauce (page 8)

Cook the spring greens in a pan of boiling water until tender, about 20 minutes. Drain well, reserving ¼ cup/60ml of the cooking water; then coarsely chop the greens and set aside. Heat the reserved cooking water in a large frying pan over medium heat. Add the onion, garlic, paprika, turmeric and Savory Spice Blend to taste. Cover and cook until the onions are soft, about 4 minutes. Stir in the miso, tomatoes, black-eyed peas, greens and Healthy Hot Sauce to taste. Simmer to heat through and combine the flavors, about 10 minutes. Serve hot.

Daily Dozen Foods

✗ BEANS   ✗ GREENS   ✗ OTHER VEGETABLES   ✗ HERBS AND SPICES

BRAISED TEMPEH & BOK CHOY WITH SPICY GINGER SAUCE

MAKES: *4* SERVINGS · DIFFICULTY: *moderate*

Although tofu is highly nutritious, I prefer tempeh as it is a *whole* soya food with fewer nutrients removed. I love it in this dish, but you can also modify this recipe with ease by skipping the tempeh and adding more bok choy or other veggies with a different bean.

16 ounces/450g tempeh, cut into ½-inch/1cm dice

1 cup/250ml Vegetable Broth (page 6) or water

1 medium red onion, chopped

3 to 4 small heads baby bok choy, trimmed and halved lengthwise, or 5 cups/500g coarsely chopped bok choy

3 garlic cloves, minced

2 tablespoons grated fresh ginger

2 tablespoons white miso paste

1 tablespoon rice vinegar

2 tablespoons Umami Sauce (page 5)

½ teaspoon chilli flakes, or to taste

1 teaspoon date sugar

½ red pepper, minced

1 cup/100g chopped mushrooms

4 spring onions, chopped

Steam the tempeh in a steamer basket over boiling water for 15 minutes. Uncover and set aside.

Heat ¼ cup/60ml of the broth in a large frying pan or wok over medium-high heat. Add the onion and bok choy, and cook, stirring until tender, about 5 minutes. Remove from the frying pan and set aside.

Heat the remaining ¾ cup/190ml of broth in the same frying pan over medium heat. Stir in the garlic, ginger, miso, vinegar, Umami Sauce, chilli flakes and date sugar. Add the pepper, mushrooms, spring onions and steamed tempeh and stir to combine. Lower the heat to a simmer and cook for 5 minutes longer, stirring occasionally. Add the onion and bok choy, and cook for about 3 minutes longer to heat through. Serve hot.

GINGER

A double-blind, randomized, controlled clinical trial compared the efficacy of ginger for the treatment of migraine headaches to sumatriptan (Imitrex), one of the top-selling drugs in the world. A pinch of powdered ginger worked just as well and just as fast as the drug[125] (and costs less than a penny). Ginger can also help with menstrual cramps, which plague up to 90 percent of younger women. Just ⅛ teaspoon of ginger powder three times a day started a few days before one's period was found to drop pain from an 8 to a 6 on a scale of 1 to 10, and down further to a 3 in the following month.[126]

Daily Dozen Foods

X BEANS   X CRUCIFEROUS VEGETABLES   X OTHER VEGETABLES   X HERBS AND SPICES

CHICKPEA & CAULIFLOWER CURRY

MAKES: *4* SERVINGS · DIFFICULTY: *easy*

This curry marries legumes and cruciferous vegetables, two of the superstar plant families, in a match made in heaven. If you aren't in the mood for green beans, substitute green peas or edamame. Serve over cooked brown rice.

1 cup/250ml Vegetable Broth (page 6)

1 red onion, chopped

2 garlic cloves, chopped

1 jalapeño pepper, seeded and minced (optional)

1½ tablespoons curry powder

1 head cauliflower, trimmed and cut into small florets

8 ounces/225g green beans, trimmed and cut into 1-inch/2.5cm pieces

1 14.5-ounce/400g BPA-free tin or Tetra Pak salt-free diced tomatoes, undrained

2 roasted red peppers (see page 9, or shop-bought), chopped

1 cup/250ml Almond Milk (page 2)

3 tablespoons nutritional yeast (or yeast flakes)

½ teaspoon smoked paprika

1½ cups/255g cooked or 1 15.5-ounce/425g BPA-free tin or Tetra Pak salt-free chickpeas, drained and rinsed

Cooked brown rice, to serve

In a large pan, heat the broth to a boil over medium-high heat. Add the onion and garlic, cover, and cook until tender, about 3 minutes. Stir in the jalapeño (if using) and curry powder; then add the cauliflower, green beans, tomatoes and roasted peppers. Cover and bring to a boil. Reduce the heat to low and simmer until the vegetables are tender, about 20 minutes.

When the veggies are tender, use a hand blender to break up some of the vegetables. Alternatively, remove up to a quarter of the solids and liquids from the pan, purée in a blender or food processor, and then return the mixture to the pan. Stir in the Almond Milk, nutritional yeast, smoked paprika and chickpeas, and cook 5 to 10 minutes longer to heat through and blend the flavors. Serve over a bed of cooked brown rice.

Daily Dozen Foods

X BEANS   X CRUCIFEROUS VEGETABLES   X OTHER VEGETABLES   X HERBS AND SPICES   X WHOLE GRAINS

LENTIL SHEPHERD'S PIE

MAKES: *4* SERVINGS · DIFFICULTY: *moderate*

Lentils can be transformed into a delicious, nutritious soup you can make in a snap. If you're feeling a little more ambitious, you can make a meal like this wonderful savory pie.

1 small red onion, chopped

1 carrot, chopped

6 ounces/175g green beans, trimmed and cut into ½-inch/1cm pieces

1 courgette or yellow (summer) squash, chopped

1 cup/250ml Vegetable Broth (page 6)

8 ounces/225g mushrooms, chopped

1 tablespoon plus 1 teaspoon white miso paste

2 tablespoons Umami Sauce (page 5)

1 teaspoon minced fresh thyme or ½ teaspoon dried

3 tablespoons nutritional yeast (or yeast flakes)

Ground black pepper

2 cups/150g cooked lentils

Cauliflower Mash (page 175)

Steam the onion, carrot and green beans in a steamer basket over boiling water for 5 minutes. Add the courgette and steam for 3 minutes longer, or until the vegetables are tender. Drain and set aside in a shallow baking dish.

Heat the broth in a saucepan over medium heat. Add the mushrooms, miso, Umami Sauce, thyme, 2 tablespoons of the nutritional yeast and black pepper to taste. Cook, stirring, for 5 minutes, or until the mushrooms are soft. Transfer to a blender or food processor. Add ½ cup/35g of the cooked lentils and blend until smooth. Add up to ½ cup/120ml of additional broth to make the gravy smoother, as desired. Combine the gravy with the remaining 1½ cups/115g of lentils, add to the steamed vegetables, and stir. Set aside.

Preheat the oven to 375°F/190°C/gas mark 5. Stir the remaining 1 tablespoon of nutritional yeast into the Cauliflower Mash; then spoon it on top of the lentils and vegetables, smoothing to cover the surface. Bake until hot, 30 to 40 minutes.

TIP: To save some time, you can substitute about 3 cups/450g of frozen mixed vegetables for the carrot, green beans and courgette. Simply steam them, and then proceed with the recipe.

Daily Dozen Foods

✗ BEANS   ✗ CRUCIFEROUS VEGETABLES   ✗ OTHER VEGETABLES   ✗ HERBS AND SPICES

YELLOW SPLIT PEA DAL
WITH WATERCRESS

MAKES: *4* SERVINGS · DIFFICULTY: *easy*

My favorite way of preparing split peas is to make a warm and comforting soup. (It's a classic for a reason.) I also throw split peas in the rice cooker, the way I prepare lentils. The following is yet another way to add these nutritious little gems into your daily diet. Remember: In my ideal world, we're all enjoying legumes (beans, chickpeas, split peas or lentils) with every meal.

If you prefer, use any type of lentil instead of the yellow split peas in this recipe. Don't have watercress? Use spinach or rocket instead. Serve this gorgeous dal over brown, black or red rice. *Dal*, by the way, is the Indian word for 'split pea', or a dish made with them.

1½ cups/300g dried yellow split peas, picked through and rinsed

3 cups/710ml Vegetable Broth (page 6) or water

3 cups/675g coarsely chopped watercress or spinach

1 14.5-ounce/400g BPA-free tin or Tetra Pak salt-free diced cherry tomatoes, drained

¼ cup/12g chopped fresh coriander

2 garlic cloves, minced

1 tablespoon finely chopped fresh ginger

1 small hot green chilli, seeded and minced

2 tablespoons nutritional yeast (or yeast flakes)

1 teaspoon white miso paste

1 teaspoon ground cumin

½ teaspoon ground coriander

1 ¼-inch/5mm piece fresh turmeric, grated (or ¼ teaspoon ground)

2 teaspoons blended peeled lemon (see page 3)

Cover the split peas with boiling water and soak for 1 hour. Drain, then transfer to a saucepan with the broth and bring to a boil. Lower the heat to a simmer and cook until the split peas are tender, 45 to 60 minutes, adding a little more broth, if needed.

When the split peas are soft, add the watercress, tomatoes and coriander, stirring to wilt the watercress. Keep warm over very low heat.

Heat 2 tablespoons of water in a small frying pan over medium heat. Add the garlic, ginger and chilli. Cook until softened, about 1 minute. Remove from the heat and add the nutritional yeast, miso, cumin, coriander, turmeric and lemon, stirring to mix well. Add the spice mixture to the split pea dal, stirring to combine. Serve hot.

Daily Dozen Foods

✗ BEANS   ✗ GREENS   ✗ OTHER VEGETABLES   ✗ HERBS AND SPICES

LOUISIANA-STYLE SOY CURLS

MAKES: *4* SERVINGS · DIFFICULTY: *easy*

Soy Curls are a shelf-stable meat substitute containing a single ingredient – whole soya beans – that are available at natural food stores or online. If you prefer, you can substitute 8 ounces/225g of steamed, diced tempeh or 1½ cups/95g of cooked or tinned dark red kidney beans.

This Creole-inspired dish is best served on a bed of cooked greens or whole grains.

1 cup/45g Soy Curls

1¼ cups/285ml Vegetable Broth (page 6) or water

1 tablespoon salt-free Creole seasoning blend

2 tablespoons jarred tomato purée

2 teaspoons white miso paste

1 large red onion, chopped

1 large green pepper, seeded and chopped

2 celery stalks, chopped

3 garlic cloves, chopped

1 14.5-ounce/400g BPA-free tin or Tetra Pak salt-free diced tomatoes, drained

2 bay leaves

1 teaspoon dried thyme

½ teaspoon dried basil

Savory Spice Blend (page 4)

Ground black pepper

Healthy Hot Sauce (page 8)

Place the Soy Curls in a large saucepan with the broth and Creole seasoning. Bring to a boil. Cover and simmer for 5 minutes. Stir in the tomato purée, miso, onion, pepper, celery and garlic. Cover and cook until the vegetables are softened, about 10 minutes. Stir in the tomatoes, bay leaves, thyme, basil, Savory Spice Blend and black pepper to taste and cook, uncovered, for about 15 minutes to blend the flavors and reduce the liquid. Remove the bay leaves before serving with Healthy Hot Sauce.

Daily Dozen Foods

X BEANS   X OTHER VEGETABLES   X HERBS AND SPICES

BEAN PATTIES WITH HARISSA

MAKES: *4* SERVINGS · DIFFICULTY: *easy*

There are dozens of ways to make delicious patties. One reason I love this recipe so much is that the patties are heartier and nuttier than most, which make for an even better meal. Rather than in a bun, serve this dish on a bed of cooked greens.

1 tablespoon ground flaxseeds (or linseeds)

2 teaspoons blended peeled lemon (see page 3)

½ cup/50g rolled oats

1½ cups/95g cooked or 1 15.5-ounce/425g BPA-free tin or Tetra Pak salt-free kidney beans or black beans, drained and rinsed

½ cup/55g chopped walnuts

½ cup/75g chopped onion

2 garlic cloves

1 ¼-inch/5mm piece fresh turmeric, grated (or ¼ teaspoon ground)

2 tablespoons tahini

2 tablespoons nutritional yeast (or yeast flakes)

1 tablespoon white miso paste

½ teaspoon smoked paprika

2 tablespoons minced fresh parsley

Harissa (page 9)

In a small bowl, combine the flaxseeds and lemon, stirring until well blended. Set aside. Grind the oats into a coarse flour in a food processor. Add the beans, walnuts, onion, garlic and turmeric and process until well combined. Add the tahini, nutritional yeast, miso, paprika, parsley and flaxseed mixture. Pulse until well combined. Shape into four patties. (They will be sticky.) Place the patties on a baking sheet lined with a silicone mat or baking parchment and refrigerate for 30 minutes. Preheat the oven to 350°F/180°C/gas mark 4. Bake the patties for 30 minutes; then flip them with a metal spatula and bake for another 15 minutes, or until firm and browned. Serve topped with Harissa.

BEANS

Researchers have found that premenopausal women who ate more than about 6 grams of soluble fiber a day (the equivalent of about a single cup/62g of black beans) had 62 percent lower odds of breast cancer compared with women who consumed less than around 4 grams a day. Meanwhile, the American Institute for Cancer Research sifted through some half a million studies and created a landmark scientific consensus report reviewed by twenty-one of the top cancer researchers in the world. One of their summary cancer prevention recommendations is to eat whole grains and/ or legumes (beans, split peas, chickpeas or lentils) with every meal.[127] Not every week or every day. *With every meal!*

Daily Dozen Foods

✗ BEANS   ✗ OTHER VEGETABLES   ✗ FLAXSEEDS   ✗ NUTS AND SEEDS   ✗ HERBS AND SPICES   ✗ WHOLE GRAINS

MAC & CHEESE

VEGETABLE UNFRIED RICE

BUCKWHEAT SOBA & EDAMAME WITH ALMOND BUTTER SAUCE

QUINOA PILAF WITH CARROTS & CHICKPEAS

WHOLE WHEAT PASTA WITH LENTIL BOLOGNESE

YELLOW RICE & BLACK BEANS WITH BROCCOLI

STUFFED WINTER SQUASH WITH BLACK BEAN SAUCE

RED QUINOA LOAF WITH GOLDEN GRAVY

HOPPIN' JOHN STUFFED SPRING GREENS ROLLS

ROCKET PESTO PASTA WITH ROASTED VEGETABLES

GREAT GRAINS

Why limit yourself to plain old white rice when there are scores of
different whole grains waiting for you to enjoy with tremendous
flavor (and many more health benefits)? Some of my favorites are
brown, red or black rice. Yes, they have longer cooking times, which
is why I often cook up large batches, portion and freeze them so I can
quickly thaw, prepare and dig in. As you look through these dishes,
keep in mind that other whole grains like barley, buckwheat, millet,
freekeh and oats can be used interchangeably in these recipes. I've
also included some fantastic whole-grain pasta options for you.

MAC & CHEESE

MAKES: *4* SERVINGS · DIFFICULTY: *easy*

Comfort food extraordinaire! If you want to make a hob version of this dish, prepare as directed, but instead of baking in the oven, combine everything except the bread crumbs and ¼ teaspoon of the smoked paprika in a pan and heat over medium heat until hot, stirring so it doesn't burn. Sprinkle on the bread crumbs, top with the smoked paprika and serve.

3 cups/710ml Vegetable Broth (page 6)

½ cup/75g chopped red onion

1 garlic clove, chopped

1½ cups/225g chopped carrot or butternut squash

8 ounces/225g 100% whole-grain or bean-based macaroni or other bite-sized pasta

½ cup/30g nutritional yeast (or yeast flakes)

2 tablespoons almond butter

2 teaspoons blended peeled lemon (see page 3)

2 teaspoons white miso paste

1 teaspoon salt-free whole-grain mustard

½ teaspoon smoked paprika

¼ teaspoon fresh turmeric, grated (or ¼ teaspoon ground)

1 teaspoon Savory Spice Blend (page 4), or to taste

1 cup/225g steamed chopped greens or small broccoli florets, liquid pressed out

¼ cup/15g whole-grain bread crumbs

In a large saucepan, heat 1 cup/250ml of the broth over medium-high heat. Add the onion, garlic and carrot. Cover and cook until the vegetables are very soft, 8 to 10 minutes. Remove from the heat and set aside.

Cook the macaroni according to the packet instructions until it is al dente. Drain well and set aside.

Preheat the oven to 375°F/190°C/gas mark 5.

In a high-speed blender, combine the cooked vegetables, the remaining 2 cups/460ml of broth, and the nutritional yeast, almond butter, lemon, miso, mustard, ¼ teaspoon of the paprika, the turmeric and Savory Spice Blend. Blend until very smooth. Taste and adjust the seasonings, if necessary.

Combine the sauce with the drained macaroni, stirring gently to combine. Stir in the cooked greens. Transfer to a 2½ quart/2.3 liter baking dish. Sprinkle with the bread crumbs and the remaining ¼ teaspoon of paprika. Bake until hot and golden on top, about 20 minutes. Serve hot.

Daily Dozen Foods

✗ CRUCIFEROUS VEGETABLES ✗ OTHER VEGETABLES ✗ NUTS AND SEEDS ✗ HERBS AND SPICES ✗ WHOLE GRAINS

VEGETABLE UNFRIED RICE

MAKES: *4* SERVINGS · DIFFICULTY: *easy*

Here's a healthy, super-easy take on a classic, and the perfect dish to make with your leftover rice and veggies. What other meal can you prepare with cold cooked rice and whichever vegetables you have on hand? You can also tailor it to suit your taste by upping (or lowering) the spice.

2 tablespoons Umami Sauce (page 5)

1 tablespoon tahini

1 teaspoon white miso paste

1 teaspoon rice vinegar

¼ to ½ teaspoon chilli flakes (optional)

1 red onion, finely chopped

1 large carrot, grated

2 cups/350g small broccoli florets

2 garlic cloves, minced

2 to 3 teaspoons grated fresh ginger

3 spring onions, minced

3 cups/750g cold cooked brown, red or black rice

1 cup/150g green peas

In a small bowl, combine the Umami Sauce, tahini, miso, vinegar and chilli flakes (if using). Stir in ¼ cup/60ml of water and set aside.

Heat ¼ cup/60ml of water in a large frying pan or wok over medium-high heat. Add the onion and carrot, and cook, stirring, until softened, about 5 minutes. Add the broccoli, garlic, ginger and spring onions and cook for 4 minutes, continuing to stir. Add the rice, peas and Umami Sauce mixture. Cook, stirring until hot and well combined, about 5 minutes. Serve immediately.

Daily Dozen Foods

✗ CRUCIFEROUS VEGETABLES   ✗ OTHER VEGETABLES   ✗ NUTS AND SEEDS   ✗ HERBS AND SPICES   ✗ WHOLE GRAINS

BUCKWHEAT SOBA & EDAMAME WITH ALMOND BUTTER SAUCE

MAKES: *4* SERVINGS · DIFFICULTY: *easy*

Buckwheat is another of my mother's favorite foods. Most mornings, she starts her day with kasha, or roasted buckwheat, as a hot cereal, and adds berries and Ceylon cinnamon. There are plenty of other uses for buckwheat as well, especially as soba noodles. (*Soba* is the Japanese term for 'buckwheat'.)

¼ cup/56g almond butter

1 garlic clove, chopped

2 teaspoons minced fresh ginger

2 tablespoons Umami Sauce (page 5)

½ teaspoon chilli flakes, or to taste

1 tablespoon blended peeled lime (see page 3)

1 tablespoon white miso paste

8 ounces/225g 100% soba noodles

1 cup/75g frozen shelled edamame, thawed

1 red pepper, cut into thin strips

1 carrot, shredded

3 spring onions, chopped

1 tablespoon sesame seeds

In a blender or food processor, combine the almond butter, garlic, ginger, Umami Sauce, chilli flakes, lime, miso and ⅔ cup/160ml of water. Blend until smooth. Set aside.

Cook the soba according to the packet instructions, adding the edamame to cook with the soba noodles. Drain and run the noodles and edamame under cold water. Transfer to a serving bowl and add the pepper, carrot and spring onions. Stir the sauce into the noodles and vegetables, tossing gently to coat. Taste and adjust the seasonings, if needed. Sprinkle with the sesame seeds and serve at room temperature.

VARIATIONS: Replace the edamame with diced cooked tempeh. Use peanut butter or tahini in place of the almond butter.

NUTS

Sometimes it feels like there just aren't enough hours in a day to get everything done. So, instead of trying to make your day longer, why not make your life longer by an extra two years? That's about how long your life span may be increased by eating nuts regularly – one handful (or about a quarter of a cup) five or more days a week.[128] Just that one simple and delicious act alone may extend your life.

Daily Dozen Foods

✗ BEANS   ✗ OTHER VEGETABLES   ✗ NUTS AND SEEDS   ✗ HERBS AND SPICES   ✗ WHOLE GRAINS

QUINOA PILAF WITH CARROTS & CHICKPEAS

MAKES: *4* SERVINGS · DIFFICULTY: *easy*

Brown, red or black rice, whole wheat couscous, or another whole grain may be used instead of the quinoa – just adjust the cooking time accordingly.

1 cup/170g quinoa, well rinsed and drained

2 teaspoons blended peeled lemon (see page 3)

1 teaspoon date sugar

1 teaspoon cumin seeds

1 teaspoon smoked paprika

1 teaspoon white miso paste

1 teaspoon Savory Spice Blend (page 4), or to taste

3 carrots, finely chopped

1½ cups/170g cooked or 1 15.5-ounce/425g BPA-free tin or Tetra Pak salt-free chickpeas, drained and rinsed

1 cup/150g peas

⅓ cup/50g raisins

¼ cup/10g minced fresh coriander or parsley

Bring 2 cups/500ml of water to a boil in a saucepan. Add the quinoa and lower the heat to a simmer. Cover and cook until the quinoa is tender and the water is absorbed, about 15 minutes. Set aside.

In a large bowl, whisk together the lemon, date sugar, cumin seeds, paprika, miso and Savory Spice Blend. Add the quinoa, carrots, chickpeas and peas and toss to coat. Add the raisins and coriander and toss again to combine. Serve immediately. Alternatively, you can serve this pilaf chilled – just cover and refrigerate for 1 to 2 hours before serving.

Daily Dozen Foods

X BEANS   X OTHER VEGETABLES   X HERBS AND SPICES   X WHOLE GRAINS

WHOLE WHEAT PASTA WITH LENTIL BOLOGNESE

MAKES: *4* SERVINGS · DIFFICULTY: *easy*

This sauce has it all – veggies, herbs, spice, protein and much more. Don't limit yourself to enjoying it only with pasta. It's delicious on a bed of cooked greens; over brown, black or red rice; or as a stuffing for peppers.

1 28-ounce/800g jar or Tetra Pak salt-free diced tomatoes, undrained

1 medium red onion, finely chopped

3 garlic cloves, minced

8 ounces/225g chestnut mushrooms, finely chopped

¼ cup/55g jarred tomato purée

1 tablespoon white miso paste

2 tablespoons nutritional yeast (or yeast flakes)

1½ teaspoons dried basil

1 teaspoon dried oregano

½ teaspoon chilli flakes

½ teaspoon date sugar

1½ cups/110g cooked or tinned lentils

8 ounces/225g 100% whole-grain or bean-based spaghetti

Nutty Parm (page 4)

Pour the liquid from the jar of tomatoes into a large frying pan over medium heat. Set the tomatoes aside for now. Add the onion and garlic and cook, stirring occasionally, until softened, about 5 minutes. Add the mushrooms and cook for 2 minutes longer; then stir in the tomato purée, miso, nutritional yeast, basil, oregano, chilli flakes and date sugar. Stir in 1 cup/250ml of water, and then add the tomatoes and lentils, and simmer, stirring frequently, for 15 minutes, or until the sauce has thickened and the flavors have blended, adding a little more water, if desired. Taste and adjust the seasonings, if needed. Keep warm over low heat.

While the sauce is simmering, cook the spaghetti in a large pan of boiling water, stirring occasionally, until it is al dente. To serve, top the pasta with the sauce and sprinkle with Nutty Parm. Serve hot.

Daily Dozen Foods

✗ BEANS   ✗ OTHER VEGETABLES   ✗ NUTS AND SEEDS   ✗ HERBS AND SPICES   ✗ WHOLE GRAINS

YELLOW RICE & BLACK BEANS WITH BROCCOLI

MAKES: *4* SERVINGS · DIFFICULTY: *easy*

If you prefer, use white beans instead of black beans. I like to add chopped tomatoes and minced spring onions just before serving for an extra oomph of color and zest.

1 large shallot, minced

1 teaspoon minced fresh ginger

2 teaspoons white miso paste

2 tablespoons nutritional yeast (or yeast flakes)

1 ¼-inch/5mm piece fresh turmeric, grated (or ¼ teaspoon ground)

½ teaspoon ground coriander

¼ teaspoon ground cumin

⅛ teaspoon cayenne pepper

1 cup/225g long-grain brown, red or black rice

2½ cups/600ml Vegetable Broth (page 6) or water

3 cups/525g small broccoli florets

1½ cups/95g cooked or 1 15.5-ounce/425g BPA-free tin or Tetra Pak salt-free black beans, drained and rinsed

Heat 2 tablespoons of water in a large frying pan or saucepan over medium-high heat. Add the shallots and ginger and cook for 1 minute. Stir in the miso, nutritional yeast, turmeric, coriander, cumin, cayenne and rice. Stir in the broth and bring to a boil. Lower the heat to a simmer, cover, and cook for 35 to 40 minutes, stirring occasionally, or until the rice is just tender. Stir in the broccoli and a little more broth, if needed. Cook for 10 minutes longer, or until the water is absorbed and the broccoli and rice are tender. Stir in the beans and remove from the heat. Serve hot.

Daily Dozen Foods

✗ BEANS   ✗ CRUCIFEROUS VEGETABLES   ✗ HERBS AND SPICES   ✗ WHOLE GRAINS

STUFFED WINTER SQUASH WITH BLACK BEAN SAUCE

MAKES: *4* SERVINGS • DIFFICULTY: *moderate*

If you can't find a squash large enough for stuffing, you can cut the squash into ½-inch/1cm-thick slices, roast them, and then arrange them in a baking dish, topped with the stuffing. Cover and bake at 350°F/180°C/gas mark 4 for 30 minutes and serve with the sauce drizzled on top.

1 large winter squash (such as buttercup or kabocha), halved and seeded

STUFFING

1 small red onion, chopped

2 cups/200g finely chopped red cabbage

2 garlic cloves, minced

1 small red, green, orange or yellow pepper, chopped

2¼ cups/530ml Vegetable Broth (page 6)

1 tablespoon white miso paste

2 tablespoons nutritional yeast (or yeast flakes)

1 cup/225g bulgur wheat

BLACK BEAN SAUCE

½ cup/120ml Vegetable Broth (page 6)

2 garlic cloves, minced

1½ cups/95g cooked or 1 15.5-ounce /425g BPA-free tin or Tetra Pak salt-free black beans, drained and rinsed

2 tablespoons Umami Sauce (page 5)

1 tablespoon white miso paste

1 tablespoon jarred tomato purée

2 tablespoons nutritional yeast (or yeast flakes)

½ teaspoon ground cumin

1 teaspoon ground coriander

⅛ to ¼ teaspoon cayenne pepper

Preheat the oven to 375°F/190°C/gas mark 5. Arrange the squash halves, cut side down, in a shallow baking tin. Add ¼ inch/5mm of water to the tin and cover tightly. Bake for 20 minutes to soften slightly.

STUFFING: Heat ¼ cup/60ml of water in a large frying pan over medium heat. Add the onion, cabbage, garlic and pepper. Cover and cook until softened, about 4 minutes. Stir in the broth, miso, nutritional yeast and bulgur. Bring to a boil, then reduce the heat to low, and simmer 5 minutes longer. Remove from the heat and let it sit, covered, for 10 minutes, or until the water is absorbed by the bulgur.

Turn over the squash halves so they are cut side up and fill them with the stuffing, packing them well. Cover and bake until the squash is tender, about 30 minutes.

SAUCE: While the stuffed squash is baking, make the sauce. In a saucepan, combine the broth and garlic and bring to a boil. Lower the heat to a simmer and stir in the beans, Umami Sauce, miso, tomato purée, nutritional yeast, cumin, coriander and cayenne. Simmer for 5 minutes; then transfer to a blender or food processor and blend until smooth, adding a little more broth, if needed, for the desired consistency. Return the sauce to the saucepan and keep warm over low heat. Taste and adjust the seasonings, if needed. To serve, top the baked squash with the sauce and serve hot.

Daily Dozen Foods

✗ BEANS   ✗ CRUCIFEROUS VEGETABLES   ✗ OTHER VEGETABLES   ✗ HERBS AND SPICES   ✗ WHOLE GRAINS

RED QUINOA LOAF
WITH GOLDEN GRAVY

MAKES: *6* SERVINGS · DIFFICULTY: *moderate*

I like to serve this dish on a bed of cooked greens. If you can't find red quinoa, look for black quinoa or, in a pinch, regular. It's also fantastic over black, red or brown rice.

QUINOA LOAF

1 small red onion, coarsely chopped

1 garlic clove, crushed

½ cup/55g walnuts

1 cup/100g mushrooms, quartered

1½ cups/95g cooked or 1 15.5-ounce/425g BPA-free tin or Tetra Pak salt-free dark red kidney beans, drained and rinsed

1 cup/170g cooked red quinoa

½ cup/50g rolled oats

2 tablespoons tahini or peanut butter

2 tablespoons nutritional yeast (or yeast flakes)

2 tablespoons ground flaxseeds (or linseeds)

1 tablespoon minced fresh parsley

1 tablespoon white miso paste

1 teaspoon smoked paprika

½ teaspoon dried thyme

½ teaspoon dried sage

½ teaspoon dried basil

¼ teaspoon ground black pepper

QUINOA LOAF: Preheat the oven to 350ºF/180ºC/gas mark 4. Line a loaf tin with a piece of baking parchment the same length of the loaf tin and long enough to come up and over the sides by an inch or two. (For an 8 × 4 × 2½-inch/20 x 10 x 6cm loaf tin, your baking parchment should be about 8 × 11 inches/20 x 27cm.)

Combine the onion, garlic and walnuts in a food processor and pulse until finely minced. Add the mushrooms and beans and pulse until finely chopped and well combined. Add the remaining loaf ingredients and process until well combined. If the mixture seems too wet to hold together, add more oats. If the mixture seems too dry, add a little water.

Transfer the mixture into the prepared loaf tin. Press firmly into the tin, smoothing the top. Bake until firm and golden brown, 50 to 60 minutes. Check at around 40 minutes: if the top of the loaf is getting too brown, cover with foil for the last 10 to 20 minutes of baking time.

Daily Dozen Foods

✗ BEANS   ✗ FLAXSEEDS   ✗ NUTS AND SEEDS   ✗ HERBS AND SPICES   ✗ WHOLE GRAINS

GOLDEN GRAVY

⅓ cup/80ml Vegetable Broth (page 6)

2 garlic cloves, minced

1½ cups/225g cooked or 1 15.5-ounce /425g BPA-free tin or Tetra Pak salt-free chickpeas, drained and rinsed

2 tablespoons nutritional yeast (or yeast flakes)

1 tablespoon white miso paste

1 teaspoon dried thyme

1 ¼-inch/5mm piece fresh turmeric, grated (or ¼ teaspoon ground)

¼ teaspoon ground black pepper

GOLDEN GRAVY: While the loaf is baking, make the gravy. In a saucepan, combine the broth and garlic and bring to a boil. Lower the heat to a simmer and stir in all the remaining gravy ingredients. Simmer for 5 minutes, and then transfer to a blender or food processor and blend until smooth. Return the gravy to the saucepan. Taste and adjust the seasonings, if needed. Keep warm over low heat.

When the loaf is done baking, remove it from the oven, uncover, and let sit for 10 minutes before slicing. Top with the gravy. Serve hot.

HOPPIN' JOHN STUFFED SPRING GREENS ROLLS

MAKES: *4* TO *6* SERVINGS (2 ROLLS PER SERVING) · DIFFICULTY: *moderate*

This Southern riff on stuffed cabbage rolls take some time to assemble, but it is more than worth the effort. For an easier variation, cook the spring greens until tender, then chop and stir them into the rice mixture, add the remaining ingredients, and heat until hot.

1 14.5-ounce/400g BPA-free tin or Tetra Pak salt-free diced tomatoes, undrained

1 red onion, minced

1 green pepper, minced

3 garlic cloves, minced

1 teaspoon smoked paprika

½ teaspoon dried thyme

¼ teaspoon cayenne pepper

¼ teaspoon ground black pepper

1½ cups/375g cooked brown, black or red rice

1½ cups/95g cooked or 1 15.5-ounce/425g BPA-free tin or Tetra Pak salt-free black-eyed peas, drained and rinsed

8 to 12 spring greens leaves, well washed, ends trimmed

1 teaspoon Healthy Hot Sauce (page 8), or to taste

2 tablespoons nutritional yeast (or yeast flakes)

1 teaspoon white miso paste

Pour the tomato liquid into a large, nonstick frying pan over medium-high heat, setting the tomatoes aside. Add the onion, cover, and cook for 3 minutes to soften. Stir in the pepper and garlic and cook 3 minutes longer or until soft, adding a little water, if needed, so they don't burn. Stir in the paprika, thyme, cayenne and black pepper. Add the cooked rice and black-eyed peas. Reduce the heat to low and cook for about 10 minutes, stirring frequently, to mix well and blend the flavors. Remove from the heat and set aside.

Bring a large pan of water to boil. Place one of the spring greens leaves, stem side up, on a flat work surface. Use a sharp knife to remove as much of the thick central rib as you can without cutting through the leaf. Repeat with the remaining leaves. Working in batches, place the spring greens leaves into the boiling water, pressing them down to keep them submerged. Boil for about 3 minutes. Remove the leaves from the pan with a slotted spoon and rinse under cool water. Preheat the oven to 350°F/180°C/gas mark 4.

In a bowl, combine the reserved diced tomatoes with the Healthy Hot Sauce, nutritional yeast and miso, stirring to blend. Spoon half of the seasoned tomatoes onto the bottom of a large, shallow baking dish and set aside. On a flat work surface, place a green leaf with its stem end nearest you. Place about 3 tablespoons of the rice mixture about a quarter of the way from the bottom of the leaf. Fold the sides of the leaf over the middle and then fold the stem end over the filling, tucking it in behind the filling. Roll up tightly and carefully place it into the baking dish. Repeat until all of the rolls are prepared. Spoon the remaining seasoned tomato mixture over the rolls. Tightly cover the baking dish and bake for 50 to 60 minutes, or until the rolls are tender. Serve hot.

Daily Dozen Foods

✗ GREENS   ✗ OTHER VEGETABLES   ✗ HERBS AND SPICES   ✗ WHOLE GRAINS

ROCKET PESTO PASTA WITH ROASTED VEGETABLES

MAKES: *4* SERVINGS · DIFFICULTY: *easy*

For a variation, omit the pasta and serve on a bed of red, black or brown rice or another one of your favorite whole grains.

3 garlic cloves

3 cups/675g fresh rocket or spinach

1 cup/30g fresh basil leaves

2 tablespoons tahini

2 tablespoons white miso

1 tablespoon brown rice vinegar

4 shallots, halved or quartered

1 large red or yellow pepper, cut into large dice

2 courgettes, trimmed and cut into ½-inch/1cm slices

8 white mushrooms

8 cherry tomatoes

¼ teaspoon onion powder

¼ teaspoon garlic powder

¼ teaspoon ground black pepper

8 ounces/225g whole-grain pasta, bean noodles, or your favorite spiralized vegetable noodles

Nutty Parm (page 4)

Chop the garlic in a food processor. Add the rocket and basil, and process until minced. Add the tahini, miso and vinegar, and continue to process until smooth and creamy. Transfer to a small bowl and set aside.

Preheat the oven to 425°F/220°C/gas mark 7. Line a large baking sheet with a silicone mat or baking parchment and set aside. Place the shallots, pepper, courgettes, mushrooms and tomatoes in a large bowl and sprinkle with the onion powder, garlic powder and black pepper, tossing to coat. Transfer the seasoned vegetables to the prepared baking sheet and place in a single layer. Roast the vegetables until tender, 20 to 25 minutes, turning once about halfway through.

While the vegetables are roasting, cook the pasta in a pan of boiling water according to the packet instructions. Drain the pasta, reserving ½ cup/120ml of the cooking liquid. Transfer the pasta to a large, shallow bowl. Blend the hot pasta liquid with the rocket pesto and add to the pasta, tossing to coat. Top with the roasted vegetables and sprinkle with Nutty Parm to taste. Serve hot.

Daily Dozen Foods

✗ GREENS ✗ OTHER VEGETABLES ✗ NUTS AND SEEDS ✗ HERBS AND SPICES ✗ WHOLE GRAINS

TEN

SIDES

If you're looking for more ways to prepare vegetables, this is the place. For greens that are loaded with flavor, try the Garlic Greens Sauté, the Indian-Style Spinach & Tomatoes or the Roasted Beetroots with Balsamic-Braised Beetroot Greens. The Cauliflower Mash is used to top the Lentil Shepherd's Pie on page 133, but it's also a great side dish in its own right. No one will ever say vegetables are boring when they try the Stuffed Sweet Potatoes with Balsamic-Date Glaze, Buffalo Cauliflower with Ranch Dressing or the Baked Onion Rings.

ROASTED ASPARAGUS WITH
YELLOW PEPPER BÉARNAISE

LEMON-ROASTED BRUSSELS SPROUTS
& CARROTS WITH PECANS

ROASTED BEETROOTS WITH
BALSAMIC-BRAISED BEETROOT GREENS

INDIAN-STYLE SPINACH & TOMATOES

RED CABBAGE SAUTÉ

CAULIFLOWER MASH

STUFFED SWEET POTATOES
WITH BALSAMIC-DATE GLAZE

GARLIC GREENS SAUTÉ

BAKED ONION RINGS

BUFFALO CAULIFLOWER
WITH RANCH DRESSING

ROASTED ASPARAGUS WITH YELLOW PEPPER BÉARNAISE

MAKES: *4* SERVINGS · DIFFICULTY: *easy*

Once you've roasted asparagus, you may never want to make it any other way. This healthy interpretation of béarnaise sauce – which is typically made with double cream, artery-clogging clarified butter and egg yolk – is also delicious over steamed broccoli, roasted cauliflower and baked sweet potatoes.

2 cups/500ml Vegetable Broth (page 6)

2 shallots, chopped

1 garlic clove, crushed

2 yellow peppers, seeded and chopped

1 teaspoon dried tarragon

2 teaspoons white miso paste

1 ¼-inch/5mm piece fresh turmeric, grated (or ¼ teaspoon ground)

3 tablespoons nutritional yeast (or yeast flakes)

1 tablespoon tarragon vinegar

2 teaspoons blended peeled lemon (see page 3)

16 to 20 ounces/450 to 560g asparagus, ends trimmed

Heat the broth in a saucepan over medium heat. Add the shallots and garlic and cook for 2 minutes to soften. Add the peppers and bring to a boil. Lower the heat to a simmer. Add the tarragon, miso and turmeric and cook for 30 minutes, or until the liquid reduces by half. Transfer to a blender. Add the nutritional yeast, vinegar and lemon, and process until smooth. Return the sauce to the pan and keep warm.

Preheat the oven to 425°F/220°C/gas mark 7. Line a large baking tin with a silicone mat or baking parchment and place the asparagus in a single layer. Roast the asparagus until it is tender, 10 to 18 minutes, depending on the thickness of the asparagus and how tender you like it. Transfer to a platter and drizzle with the sauce.

Daily Dozen Foods

X OTHER VEGETABLES   X HERBS AND SPICES

LEMON-ROASTED BRUSSELS SPROUTS & CARROTS WITH PECANS

MAKES: *4* SERVINGS · DIFFICULTY: *easy*

Roasting dramatically improves the flavor of Brussels sprouts. They're even better with the addition of carrots for color, pecans for crunch and a spritz of lemon to brighten the taste.

1 pound/450g Brussels sprouts, trimmed and halved lengthwise

2 carrots, cut diagonally into ¼-inch/5mm slices

2 teaspoons Savory Spice Blend (page 4)

⅓ cup/35g raw pecan pieces

1 tablespoon blended peeled lemon (see page 3)

Preheat the oven to 425°F/220°C/gas mark 7. Line a large baking tin with a silicone mat or baking parchment and place the Brussels sprouts and carrots in a single layer. Season the vegetables with half of the Savory Spice Blend and roast for 10 minutes. Remove from the oven, stir the vegetables and then roast for another 5 minutes, or until the vegetables are tender. Remove from the oven once again. Transfer to a platter and sprinkle with the pecans, lemon and remaining spice blend.

BRUSSELS SPROUTS

Consuming Brussels sprouts (along with cabbage, cauliflower and broccoli) has been associated with a lower risk of colon cancer in the middle and right side of your body.[129] In vitro, Brussels sprout extracts were found to effectively suppress breast cancer cell growth.[130] Quite a lot of goodness in such a tiny little crucifer!

Daily Dozen Foods

✗ CRUCIFEROUS VEGETABLES   ✗ OTHER VEGETABLES   ✗ NUTS AND SEEDS   ✗ HERBS AND SPICES

ROASTED BEETROOTS WITH BALSAMIC-BRAISED BEETROOT GREENS

MAKES: *4* SERVINGS · DIFFICULTY: *easy*

Beetroots are a concentrated source of vegetable nitrates, which can lower blood pressure and improve blood flow. If you've never been a fan of beetroot, it may be because you've never had them roasted. The cooking of beetroot greens with their roots seems almost like a violation of the biblical prohibition against boiling a kid in its mother's milk, but I think we're cool.

1 bunch medium beetroots with greens

1 red onion, cut into ½-inch/1cm wedges

1 teaspoon dried oregano

½ cup/120ml balsamic vinegar

2 teaspoons date sugar

1 teaspoon grated orange zest

Ground black pepper

Preheat the oven to 400°F/200°C/gas mark 6. Remove the greens from the beetroots, rinse them well, remove and discard any large stems and set aside. Trim the ends of the beetroots, leaving the skins on, and scrub the beetroots well. If any of the beetroots are large, cut them in half lengthwise. (The beetroots should be about the same size so as to cook evenly.)

Line a large baking dish with a silicone mat or baking parchment and place the beetroots and onions in a single layer. Season with the oregano and cover tightly. Roast the vegetables for 30 minutes, then uncover, stir, and return the vegetables to the oven, uncovered, to roast for 10 minutes longer, or until the beetroots are tender when pierced with a fork.

Finely chop the beetroot greens and transfer to a frying pan with ¼ cup/60ml of water. Cook over medium heat, stirring, until the greens are just tender, about 3 minutes. Stir in the balsamic vinegar and date sugar. Increase the heat to medium-high and cook until the vinegar has reduced to a syrup consistency. Remove from the heat.

Remove the vegetables from the oven. Cut the beetroots into wedges and pull away and discard the outer skin. Transfer the beetroots and onion to a serving dish, top with the balsamic greens, and add the orange zest, tossing lightly to coat. Sprinkle with black pepper to taste and serve.

Daily Dozen Foods

X GREENS   X OTHER VEGETABLES   X HERBS AND SPICES

BEETROOT

In one study, men and women eating 1½ cups/300g of baked beetroots seventy-five minutes before running a race improved their running performance while maintaining the same heart rate and even reported less exertion.[131] Not trying to improve your splits? Keep loading up on beetroots, because a 2015 study found that people who consumed a cup/250ml of beetroot juice daily for four weeks reduced their systolic blood pressure by about 8 points.[132]

INDIAN-STYLE SPINACH & TOMATOES

MAKES: *4* SERVINGS · DIFFICULTY: *easy*

This simple recipe is bursting with flavor. It's great served over quinoa, black, red or brown rice, or even more greens.

1 pound/450g fresh spinach

1 14.5-ounce/400g BPA-free tin or Tetra Pak salt-free diced tomatoes, undrained

8 to 12 ounces/225 to 350g chestnut mushrooms, sliced

1½ teaspoons grated fresh ginger

1 teaspoon ground coriander

1 ¼-inch/5mm piece fresh turmeric, grated (or ¼ teaspoon ground)

¼ teaspoon ground cumin

¼ teaspoon chilli flakes

1 tablespoon white miso paste

Steam the spinach until tender, 3 to 5 minutes. Drain well, pressing out any excess liquid. Set aside the tomatoes for now. Purée the spinach in a blender or food processor and set aside. Drain the tomato liquid into a large frying pan over medium heat. Add the mushrooms, ginger, coriander, turmeric, cumin and chilli flakes and cook, stirring, for 1 minute. Stir in the tomatoes and miso and cook for 3 minutes before stirring in the puréed spinach. Continue cooking until the mixture is hot and well blended.

Daily Dozen Foods

✗ GREENS   ✗ OTHER VEGETABLES   ✗ HERBS AND SPICES

RED CABBAGE SAUTÉ

MAKES: *4* SERVINGS · DIFFICULTY: *easy*

This cabbage dish is especially good served over braised tempeh.

¼ cup/60ml Vegetable Broth (page 6) or water

1 medium red onion, minced

6 cups/600g finely shredded red cabbage

2 cups/200g chopped mushrooms (any variety)

2 teaspoons minced fresh thyme, or 1 teaspoon dried

3 tablespoons Umami Sauce (page 5)

Ground black pepper

Heat the broth in a medium frying pan over medium heat. Add the onion and cabbage and cook, stirring frequently, until the vegetables have softened, about 4 minutes. Add the mushrooms and thyme. Continue to cook, stirring, for about 4 more minutes. Season with the Umami Sauce, tossing to coat. Serve hot sprinkled with black pepper to taste.

Daily Dozen Foods

✗ CRUCIFEROUS VEGETABLES   ✗ OTHER VEGETABLES   ✗ HERBS AND SPICES

CAULIFLOWER MASH

MAKES: *4* SERVINGS · DIFFICULTY: *easy*

Enjoy this delightful dish in place of mashed white potatoes or as a topping for the Lentil Shepherd's Pie on page 133.

1 head cauliflower, trimmed and cut into 1-inch/2.5cm pieces

1 tablespoon nutritional yeast (or yeast flakes)

1 teaspoon white miso paste

2 teaspoons Roasted Garlic (page 6) (optional)

Steam the cauliflower until soft, about 10 minutes. Transfer to a bowl or a food processor. Add the nutritional yeast, miso and Roasted Garlic (if using) and mash or purée until smooth. Serve hot.

Daily Dozen Foods

✗ CRUCIFEROUS VEGETABLES   ✗ OTHER VEGETABLES

STUFFED SWEET POTATOES WITH BALSAMIC-DATE GLAZE

MAKES: *4* SERVINGS · DIFFICULTY: *easy*

I love sweet potatoes, one of the healthiest foods on the planet. The purple ones are the best, and you can usually find them at Asian markets and specialty natural groceries. They're so good I send them out in the mail as holiday gifts. After all, what is more comforting on a wintry day than a nice, warm, steamy sweet potato? Here's a recipe for a stocking stuffer you can stuff.

4 medium sweet potatoes

½ cup/75g green peas, steamed

2 tablespoons minced fresh chives or spring onions

¼ cup/25g raw flaked almonds

Balsamic-Date Glaze (page 8)

Ground black pepper

Preheat the oven to 400°F/200°C/gas mark 6. Place the sweet potatoes on a baking sheet lined with a silicone mat or baking parchment. Prick each potato with a fork in two or three places and bake until tender, about 1 hour.

When the potatoes are done baking, transfer them to a work surface and allow to cool slightly. Cut each sweet potato in half lengthwise and scoop out the insides of the potatoes into a bowl, leaving about ¼ inch/5mm of potato attached to the skin. Add the peas and chives and mix well. Spoon the mixture into each half and return the stuffed sweet potatoes to the oven for about 15 minutes to heat through. Sprinkle with almonds, drizzle with Balsamic-Date Glaze, add a few grinds of black pepper to taste, and serve hot.

PEAS

Like edamame, raw English peas (also known as shell or garden peas) can be a great au naturel snack. I fell in love with peas in the pod when I first picked them off the vine at a farm my brother and I spent time on one summer as kids. They were like candy. Every year, I look forward to the few weeks I can find them fresh. The rest of the year, sugar snap peas can substitute as a good vegetable finger food.

Daily Dozen Foods

✗ OTHER VEGETABLES   ✗ NUTS AND SEEDS

GARLIC GREENS SAUTÉ

MAKES: *4* SERVINGS · DIFFICULTY: *easy*

If you wish, transform this recipe into a main dish by adding about 2 cups/125g of cooked white beans and serving over quinoa or black, red or brown rice, or tossing with 100% whole-grain or bean pasta.

⅓ cup/80ml Vegetable Broth (page 6) or water

3 to 4 garlic cloves, minced

1 teaspoon dried basil

½ teaspoon dried oregano

¼ to ½ teaspoon chilli flakes

2 teaspoons white miso paste

10 to 12 ounces/300 to 350g dark leafy greens, tough stems removed, then chopped

Ground black pepper

Combine the broth, garlic, basil, oregano and chilli flakes in a large pan and bring to a boil over medium-high heat. Lower the heat to medium and cook for 1 minute to soften the garlic. Stir in the miso and then add the greens, cooking until they wilt, 2 to 6 minutes depending on the type of greens. Serve hot sprinkled with black pepper to taste.

TEN WAYS TO ENJOY GREENS

1. Add raw greens (kale, spinach) to a smoothie.
2. Sauté them (chard, kale, rocket, endive, spinach) with garlic, raisins or nuts.
3. Add them (chard, spinach, Asian greens, rocket) to a soup.
4. Steam and top them (kale, spinach) with a sauce.
5. Bake them (kale) into chips.
6. Pair them (chard, spring greens, spinach, watercress) with beans and whole grains or pasta.
7. Purée them (spinach, watercress, rocket) into a dip or sauce.
8. Add them (spinach, watercress) to a sandwich or salad.
9. Braise them (spring greens, kale) and drizzle with balsamic vinegar.
10. Stir-fry them (Asian greens, rocket, kale) with ginger and sesame seeds.

Daily Dozen Foods

✗ GREENS ✗ HERBS AND SPICES

BAKED ONION RINGS

MAKES: *4* SERVINGS (5 ONION RINGS PER SERVING) • DIFFICULTY: *moderate*

Onion rings were a favorite of mine growing up, but I thankfully (and heartfully) gave up my taste for those greasy, oily, deep-fried, fatty monstrosities. The onion rings in this recipe come out pretty close to perfection. Try them with Black Bean Burgers (page 88) and Beetroot Burgers (98).

1 large red onion, cut into ½-inch/1cm-thick slices

⅔ cup/65g oat flour

¼ cup/23g chickpea flour

1 cup/250ml Almond Milk (page 2)

1 teaspoon rice vinegar

⅓ cup/50g fine cornmeal

¾ cup/95g 100% whole-grain salt-free bread crumbs

⅓ cup/20g nutritional yeast (or yeast flakes)

2 tablespoons Savory Spice Blend (page 4)

1 teaspoon smoked paprika

Preheat the oven to 425°F/220°C/gas mark 7. Line a large baking sheet with a silicone mat or baking parchment and set aside. Separate the onion slices into rings. Transfer to a bowl and set aside.

In a shallow bowl, combine the oat flour, chickpea flour, Almond Milk and vinegar, stirring to blend well.

In a separate shallow bowl, combine the cornmeal, bread crumbs, nutritional yeast, Savory Spice Blend and paprika, mixing well.

In a row, line up the bowls of onion rings, batter and breading mixture, and the prepared baking sheet. Dip an onion ring into the batter, coating it all over. Transfer the onion ring to the breading, tossing to coat. Use a clean, dry hand to sprinkle the breading onto the onion as needed. Place the coated onion ring on the prepared baking sheet and repeat with the remaining ingredients, arranging the rings in a single layer. Use a second baking sheet, if needed. You should have enough batter and breading for about twenty onion rings. Bake for 10 minutes; then remove from the oven and carefully turn over the rings. Bake for about 10 minutes longer, or until crisp and nicely browned. Serve hot.

ONIONS

Colorectal cancer starts out as a polyp, which grows from the inner surface of the colon. A 2006 study found that six months of consuming a phytonutrient called quercetin, which is found in vegetables such as red onions, along with curcumin, an active ingredient of the spice turmeric, were found to decrease the number and size of polyps by more than half among patients with a hereditary form of colorectal cancer.[133] Eating onion along with garlic has also been associated with a significantly lower risk of prostate enlargement (known as BPH).[134]

Daily Dozen Foods

✗ BEANS   ✗ OTHER VEGETABLES   ✗ HERBS AND SPICES   ✗ WHOLE GRAINS

BUFFALO CAULIFLOWER WITH RANCH DRESSING

MAKES: *4* SERVINGS · DIFFICULTY: *moderate*

This is a fun and delicious way to enjoy one of my favorite crucifers.

½ cup/45g chickpea flour

1 tablespoon nutritional yeast (or yeast flakes)

1 teaspoon garlic powder

1 teaspoon Savory Spice Blend (page 4)

1 head cauliflower, cut into bite-sized pieces

⅔ cup/150ml Healthy Hot Sauce (page 8)

Ranch Dressing (page 7)

Preheat the oven to 425°F/220°C/gas mark 7. Line one or two large baking sheets with a silicone mat or baking parchment and set aside.

In a large bowl, combine the flour, nutritional yeast, garlic powder and Savory Spice Blend. Stream in ½ cup/120ml of water and whisk until smooth. Add the cauliflower to the batter, turning to coat each piece. Arrange the battered cauliflower on the prepared baking sheets. (Do not let them touch.) Bake for 15 minutes, turning halfway through.

Pour the Healthy Hot Sauce in a large bowl. When the cauliflower is done, remove it from the oven and gently toss it in the hot sauce. Return the cauliflower pieces to the baking sheet. Bake for 20 to 25 minutes longer, or until they become crispy. Allow to cool for 10 minutes before serving with a side of Ranch Dressing.

Daily Dozen Foods

✗ BEANS   ✗ CRUCIFEROUS VEGETABLES   ✗ NUTS AND SEEDS   ✗ HERBS AND SPICES   ✗ WHOLE GRAINS

ELEVEN

SWEETS

You only need refined flour, sugar, eggs and dairy to make sweet treats if you
want desserts that will wreak havoc with your health. Using date sugar and
date syrup as sweeteners, blending ground flaxseeds with warm water to
replace eggs and grinding rolled oats into flour are just a few of the
secrets to making delicious, decadent, whole-food desserts.

For a quick sweet nibble, try the No-Bake Oatmeal Walnut Cookies.
For a home-style dessert, dig into Baked Apple Crumbles, Two-Berry Pie
with Pecan-Sunflower Crust and Raspberry-Peach Crisp. Get your chocolate
fix with Berry Chocolate Chia Pudding, Almond-Chocolate Truffles and
Fudgy No-Bake Brownies. What about a homemade soft-serve ice-cream-y
type of dessert? It's as near as the frozen bananas in your freezer.

ALMOND-CHOCOLATE TRUFFLES

NO-BAKE OATMEAL WALNUT COOKIES

BAKED APPLE CRUMBLES

FRESH FRUIT SKEWERS WITH
BLACKBERRY COULIS

RASPBERRY-PEACH CRISP

STRAWBERRY-BANANA NICE CREAM

FUDGY NO-BAKE BROWNIES

BERRY CHOCOLATE CHIA PUDDING

TWO-BERRY PIE WITH
PECAN-SUNFLOWER CRUST

ALMOND-CHOCOLATE TRUFFLES

MAKES: ABOUT *24* · DIFFICULTY: *easy*

I've always had a sweet tooth, and the best way I can satisfy it is with fresh fruits like mangoes or dried fruits like dates. If you're going to have something sweet, you might as well make it something that's also nutritious.

⅓ cup/60g chopped and pitted soft dates

⅓ cup/50g raw cashews, soaked in hot water for 3 hours and then drained

3 tablespoons almond butter

½ cup/50g unsweetened cocoa powder

¼ cup/60g date sugar

1 2- to 3-inch/5 to 8cm piece vanilla pod, split and scraped (or 1 teaspoon extract)

Ground almonds, for coating

Combine the dates and cashews in a food processor and process to a paste. Add the almond butter and process to combine. Add the cocoa powder, date sugar, vanilla and 1 teaspoon of water. Pulse until well combined.

Pinch some of the mixture between your fingers to see whether it holds together. If it's too dry, add a little more water, 1 teaspoon at a time, until the mixture can be shaped into balls. If the mixture is too soft, refrigerate it for 20 minutes or longer to firm up. If it's still too soft, add a little more cocoa powder, 1 teaspoon at a time.

Use your hands to shape and roll a small amount of the mixture into a 1-inch/2.5cm ball and transfer to a plate. Repeat until all the mixture has been rolled into balls.

Place the ground almonds in a shallow bowl. Roll the truffles in the almonds until they're coated, pressing on them if needed to cover completely. Transfer the coated truffles to a plate and refrigerate until firm before serving.

NOTE: If your dates are not soft, soak them in hot water for 20 minutes; then drain and pat dry before using.

Daily Dozen Foods

✗ OTHER FRUITS   ✗ NUTS AND SEEDS

NO-BAKE OATMEAL WALNUT COOKIES

MAKES: *24* COOKIES · DIFFICULTY: *easy*

These delicious treats can be assembled in minutes. Then simply pop them in the fridge to firm up before devouring.

1½ cups/260g soft, pitted dates

1 cup/115g walnut pieces

1 cup/100g rolled oats

2 tablespoons date sugar, or to taste

1 tablespoon ground flaxseeds (or linseeds) blended with 2 tablespoons warm water

1 2- to 3-inch/5 to 8cm piece vanilla pod, split and scraped (or 1 teaspoon extract)

1 teaspoon ground cinnamon

Line a baking sheet with a silicone mat or baking parchment and set aside. In a food processor, combine the dates, walnuts and oats and process until crumbly. Add the date sugar, flax mixture, vanilla and cinnamon and process until the dough holds together. If the mixture is too dry to hold together, add a little water, 1 tablespoon at a time. Scoop out about 1 tablespoon of the dough and roll it between your hands to form a ball. Repeat until all the dough is used. Arrange the balls on the prepared baking sheet, spaced liberally. Use a fork to press them down to flatten slightly and make a crisscross pattern. Refrigerate for 4 hours to firm up before serving.

Daily Dozen Foods

𝗫 OTHER FRUITS   𝗫 FLAXSEEDS   𝗫 NUTS AND SEEDS   𝗫 HERBS AND SPICES   𝗫 WHOLE GRAINS

BAKED APPLE CRUMBLES

MAKES: *4* SERVINGS · DIFFICULTY: *easy*

These baked apples have all the flavor (and wonderful fragrance) of apple pie, but are much better for you.

¼ cup/30g finely chopped raw walnuts

¼ cup/25g rolled oats

1 tablespoon raisins

1 tablespoon almond butter

1 teaspoon ground cinnamon

4 large firm baking apples, washed and cored

1 teaspoon blended peeled lemon (see page 3)

1 tablespoon Date Syrup (page 3)

Preheat the oven to 350°F/180°C/gas mark 4. In a food processor, combine the walnuts, oats, raisins, almond butter and cinnamon. Pulse until well mixed. Set the crumbled mixture aside.

Peel the apples about a quarter of the way down from the top. Rub the exposed part of the apples with the lemon to prevent discoloration. Stuff the crumble mixture into the center of the cored apples. Spoon the Date Syrup on top of the crumble mixture, dividing evenly. Arrange the apples upright in a shallow baking dish and pour ½ cup/120ml of water around them. Cover and bake until tender, about 1 hour. Serve warm.

VARIATION: If you want to save time, you can 'bake' the apples in a microwave oven. Proceed as above; then arrange the apples in a microwave-safe baking dish. Microwave, uncovered, on high power until the apples are tender, 5 to 8 minutes, or longer, depending on the power of your microwave. Set aside to cool for 5 minutes before serving as the apples will be very hot inside.

APPLES

'An apple a day keeps the oncologist away.' This was the title of a study published in the *Annals of Oncology* that set out to determine whether eating an apple (or more) a day was associated with lower cancer risk. The results: compared with people who average less than one apple a day, daily apple eaters had 24 percent lower odds of breast cancer, as well as significantly lower risks for ovarian cancer, laryngeal cancer, and colorectal cancer.[135]

FRESH FRUIT SKEWERS
WITH BLACKBERRY COULIS

MAKES: *4* SERVINGS · DIFFICULTY: *easy*

This is an easy, elegant and fun way to enjoy fresh fruit. Mix and match the types of fruit depending on what's in season.

2 cups/250g blackberries

½ teaspoon blended peeled lemon (see page 3)

Date sugar

1 cup/125g hulled strawberries or raspberries

½ pineapple, peeled, cored and cut into 1½-inch/4cm chunks

1 cup/100g seedless red grapes

2 kiwi fruit, peeled and quartered

3 plums or peaches, halved, pitted and cut into 1½-inch/4cm chunks

In a food processor or blender, combine the blackberries, lemon and date sugar to taste, and process until smooth. Cover and refrigerate the coulis until needed.

Thread one piece of each type of fruit onto a skewer, adding additional fruit, depending on the length of your skewers. Arrange the skewered fruit on a platter and serve with the coulis, either drizzled on the fruit or served on the side in small bowls.

BERRIES

Berries aren't just one of the most important foods you can eat – they're also one of the most delicious. I buy big bags of them frozen so I never have to worry about whether or not they're in season. I even started growing them. The elderberry bush in our backyard is now taller than I am. The healthiest common fresh berries are probably blackberries, but I'm always on the lookout for local pick-your-own black raspberries.

Daily Dozen Foods

X BERRIES   X OTHER FRUITS

RASPBERRY-PEACH CRISP

MAKES: *6* SERVINGS · DIFFICULTY: *easy*

I'm a fan of eating seasonally whenever I can. Why not change up the fruit in this recipe according to what's in season?

TOPPING

1 cup/100g rolled oats

½ cup/55g raw pecans

¼ cup/45g pitted dates

¼ cup/60g date sugar

½ teaspoon ground cinnamon

FILLING

¼ cup/38g raw cashews, soaked in hot water for 3 hours, then drained

4 cups/900g sliced peaches

⅓ cup/80g date sugar, or more to taste

1 teaspoon blended peeled lemon (see page 3)

1 2 to 3-inch/5 to 8cm piece vanilla pod, split and scraped (or 1 teaspoon extract)

1½ cups/190g raspberries

TOPPING: In a food processor, combine the oats, pecans and dates, and pulse until finely ground. Add 2 tablespoons of water, date sugar and cinnamon and pulse until the mixture is well combined and crumbly. Set aside. Preheat the oven to 350°F/180°C/gas mark 4.

FILLING: In a high-speed blender, combine 2 tablespoons of water with the cashews, 1 cup/225g of peach slices, date sugar, lemon and vanilla and blend until smooth. In an 8-inch/20cm square baking tin or shallow baking dish, combine the remaining 3 cups/675g of peaches with the raspberries. Pour the mixture from the blender over the fruit, mixing gently to combine and spread evenly.

Crumble the topping over the fruit. Bake for 25 to 30 minutes, or until the topping begins to brown and the filling is bubbling. Allow to cool for a few minutes before serving.

Daily Dozen Foods

✗ OTHER FRUITS   ✗ NUTS AND SEEDS   ✗ WHOLE GRAINS

STRAWBERRY-BANANA NICE CREAM

MAKES: *4* SERVINGS · DIFFICULTY: *easy*

I scream, you scream, we all scream for NICE cream! We can't get enough of this dessert in our household – both this specific recipe and easy-to-make, delicious variations. Here are four other favorites:

PEANUT BUTTER-BANANA: Omit the strawberries and use peanut butter instead of almond butter.

CHOCOLATEY BANANA: Instead of the strawberries, add cocoa powder for a healthy chocolate nice cream that tastes like a banana split.

VERY CHERRY: Replace the strawberries with fresh or frozen pitted cherries.

MATCHA: Simply blend two ingredients – powdered matcha green tea and blended frozen bananas – before freezing. (Please make sure the matcha is sourced from Japan, not China, due to lead contamination concerns.)

---

4 frozen overripe bananas, broken into chunks before freezing

2 tablespoons almond butter

1 cup/200g sliced strawberries

1 1- to 1½-inch/2.5 to 4cm piece vanilla pod, split and scraped (or ½ teaspoon extract)

Combine the bananas and almond butter in a food processor and blend until smooth and creamy. Add the strawberries and vanilla and pulse to mix well, leaving a few solid bits of strawberry throughout. Transfer the nice cream to an airtight container and freeze for 30 minutes for a soft texture or for 1 to 2 hours for a firmer texture. If the nice cream becomes too hard to scoop, let it stand at room temperature for 10 to 15 minutes before serving.

TIP: Keep a stash of ripe banana chunks in the freezer to make delicious soft-serve nice cream (and smoothies) in minutes.

Daily Dozen Foods

✗ BERRIES   ✗ OTHER FRUITS   ✗ NUTS AND SEEDS

FUDGY NO-BAKE BROWNIES

MAKES: *16* (2-INCH/5CM) SQUARE BROWNIES · DIFFICULTY: *easy*

A quick and easy way to satisfy your sweet tooth while keeping it healthy.

1 cup/115g walnuts

1⅓ cups/235g dates, pitted

½ cup/110g almond butter

½ cup/50g unsweetened cocoa powder

⅓ cup/38g crushed pecans

Grind the walnuts and dates in a food processor until finely ground. Add the almond butter and process until well mixed. Add the cocoa powder and pulse to mix well.

Transfer the brownie mixture to an 8-inch/20cm square baking tin. (If you line the tin with baking parchment, it will make it easier to remove the brownies.) Use your fingers to press the mixture evenly into the tin. (You can place a piece of baking parchment on top of the mixture as you press it into the tin to prevent it from sticking to your hands.) Once the brownies are firmly pressed into the tin, sprinkle the top evenly with the crushed pecans, pressing them into the top of the brownies. Cover and refrigerate for at least 1 hour before cutting into squares.

Daily Dozen Foods

X OTHER FRUITS   X NUTS AND SEEDS

✕ BERR

BERRY CHOCOLATE CHIA PUDDING

MAKES: *4* SERVINGS · DIFFICULTY: *easy*

Avocado and almond butter add richness to this chocolaty pudding.

½ ripe Hass avocado, halved and pitted

1¼ cups/250g strawberries, blueberries, or other berries of choice

3 tablespoons unsweetened cacao powder

2 tablespoons almond butter

½ cup/120ml Date Syrup (page 3)

1½ cups/360ml Almond Milk (page 2)

¼ cup/40g chia seeds

Optional garnishes: fresh berries, raw flaked almonds, cacao nibs

Scoop out the flesh from the avocado and place it in a high-speed blender or food processor. Add the berries, cacao powder, almond butter, Date Syrup and Almond Milk. Blend until completely smooth and then pour into a bowl. Whisk in the chia seeds until they're evenly distributed. Cover and refrigerate for at least 8 hours. Divide the pudding among four small dessert bowls, garnish as desired, and refrigerate for 20 minutes before serving.

TWO-BERRY PIE WITH PECAN-SUNFLOWER CRUST

MAKES: *8* SERVINGS · DIFFICULTY: *easy*

An easy, three-ingredient crust is the base for this delicious pie with a creamy layer of filling and a fresh berry topping.

CRUST

1 cup/115g pecans or walnuts

¾ cup/98g sunflower seeds

½ cup/88g soft, pitted Medjool dates

FILLING

¾ cup/112g cashews, soaked for 3 hours in hot water, then drained

2 tablespoons date sugar

½ teaspoon blended peeled lemon (see page 3)

1 1- to 1½-inch/2.5 to 4cm piece vanilla pod, split and scraped (or ½ teaspoon extract)

½ ripe banana

1¼ cups/125g fresh blueberries, or thawed frozen

1 cup/125g fresh blackberries or small strawberries, or thawed frozen

CRUST: Combine all three of the crust ingredients in a food processor and process until coarsely ground. If the mixture doesn't hold together when pinched, add 1 to 2 tablespoons of water. Press the crust mixture into a 9-inch/23cm pie plate (lined with cling film for easy removal, if desired) or springform tin and set aside. Refrigerate the crust while you prepare the filling.

FILLING: Blend the drained cashews, date sugar, lemon and vanilla in a high-speed blender and blend until smooth. Add the banana and ½ cup/50g of the blueberries, and blend until smooth and creamy. Spread the filling evenly on top of the crust.

Arrange the blackberries and remaining ¾ cup/75g of blueberries in concentric circles on top of the filling. Refrigerate for 4 hours to firm up before serving. For best results, serve this pie on the same day it is made.

Daily Dozen Foods

✗ BERRIES   ✗ OTHER FRUITS   ✗ NUTS AND SEEDS

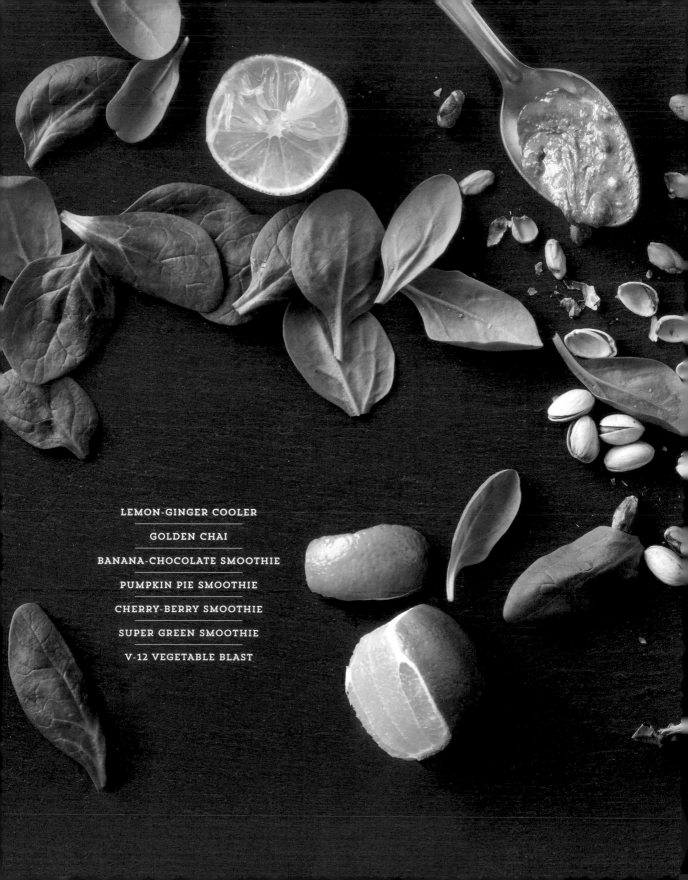

LEMON-GINGER COOLER

GOLDEN CHAI

BANANA-CHOCOLATE SMOOTHIE

PUMPKIN PIE SMOOTHIE

CHERRY-BERRY SMOOTHIE

SUPER GREEN SMOOTHIE

V-12 VEGETABLE BLAST

SIPS

Smoothie fans will enjoy the selection we've put together, ranging from Super Green to a decadent-tasting Banana-Chocolate. The Cherry-Berry Smoothie tastes like summer, and the Pumpkin Pie Smoothie is perfect for the fall and winter. If I had to pick just one, my favorite new concoction is the V-12 Vegetable Blast.

LEMON-GINGER COOLER

MAKES: *2* (2-CUP/500ML) SERVINGS · DIFFICULTY: *easy*

You can also serve this scintillating beverage as a hot tea.

1 2-inch/5cm piece fresh ginger, sliced

2 tablespoons blended peeled lemon (see page 3)

1 4-inch/10cm piece cinnamon stick (optional)

Date Syrup (page 3) (optional)

Mint sprigs, for serving (optional)

Combine 4 cups/950ml of water with the ginger in a large saucepan and bring to a boil. Remove from the heat. Add the lemon and cinnamon stick (if using) and set aside for 30 minutes. Sweeten to taste with Date Syrup (if using). Refrigerate until chilled. Serve in tall glasses over ice. Add a sprig of mint if you're in the mood.

5 WAYS TO PEP UP YOUR WATER

Add any of the following to a glass or jug of water to make a good thing even better:

1. Lemon or lime slices
2. Cucumber slices
3. Ginger slices
4. Mint leaves
5. Ice cubes with fresh berries frozen inside

Daily Dozen Foods

✗ OTHER FRUITS   ✗ HERBS AND SPICES   ✗ BEVERAGES

GOLDEN CHAI

MAKES: *4* (1½-CUP/360ML) SERVINGS · DIFFICULTY: *easy*

Turmeric adds a touch of gold to this fragrant tea that can be served hot or cold.

2 2-inch/5cm pieces cinnamon stick

1 1-inch/2.5cm piece fresh ginger, cut into thin rounds

8 whole cloves

4 green cardamom pods, smashed

2 teaspoons fennel seeds

1 ¼-inch/5mm piece fresh turmeric, grated (or ¼ teaspoon ground)

6 cups/1.4 liters cold water

6 bags Darjeeling or other black tea

¼ cup/60ml Date Syrup (page 3), or to taste

1 cup/250ml Almond Milk (page 2), or to taste

In a medium saucepan, combine the cinnamon, ginger, cloves, cardamom, fennel seeds and turmeric. Add the water and bring to a boil. Reduce the heat to low and simmer for 10 minutes. Remove from the heat. Add the tea bags and steep for 5 minutes. Remove and discard the tea bags. Stir in the Date Syrup and Almond Milk. Strain the chai into a teapot and serve.

Daily Dozen Foods

✗ OTHER FRUITS   ✗ NUTS AND SEEDS   ✗ HERBS AND SPICES   ✗ BEVERAGES

BANANA-CHOCOLATE SMOOTHIE

MAKES: *1* (2-CUP/500ML) SERVING · DIFFICULTY: *easy*

This creamy, chocolaty smoothie tastes so rich and delicious, you'll forget how healthy it is!

1 frozen ripe banana, cut into chunks before freezing

⅓ cup/35g frozen blueberries

2 tablespoons unsweetened cocoa powder

1 tablespoon ground flaxseeds (or linseeds)

1 1- to 1½-inch/2.5 to 4cm piece vanilla pod, split and scraped (or ½ teaspoon extract)

1 tablespoon almond butter

2 tablespoons Date Syrup (page 3) (optional, depending on the sweetness of the fruit)

1 cup/225g raw spinach leaves

3 to 4 ice cubes (optional)

Combine all the ingredients with 1 cup/250ml of water in a high-speed blender. Blend until thick and smooth. For a thinner texture, add less ice (if using) or more water. Serve immediately.

SMOOTHIES

My smoothie strategy is to combine super-tasty foods with those that are less tasty, such as mangoes with raw kale, so they balance each other out. Smoothies let you consume foods you might not otherwise pack into your daily diet, and they're convenient. For me, this means I can be at my treadmill desk, exercising, working, and getting some of my Daily Dozen through a straw, all at the same time!

Some people have said that when you put veggies and fruit into a blender, the fiber is somehow lost. That's ridiculous. As much fiber as goes into the blender, comes out of the blender. What a good blender can do is break down fruit and vegetable cell walls better than our teeth, and this helps release more nutrition than we would get otherwise. To avoid feeling hungry after a smoothie, though, sip smoothies slowly so that your mind and body have time to register the intake and send appropriate fullness signals.

Daily Dozen Foods

✗ BERRIES ✗ OTHER FRUITS ✗ GREENS ✗ FLAXSEEDS ✗ NUTS AND SEEDS ✗ BEVERAGES

PUMPKIN PIE SMOOTHIE

MAKES: *1* (1½-CUP/360ML) SERVING · DIFFICULTY: *easy*

This drink tastes just like pumpkin pie in a glass. Make sure you use pure pumpkin purée and not pumpkin pie filling.

½ cup/110g pure pumpkin purée

1 small frozen ripe banana, cut into chunks before freezing

3 soft Medjool dates, pitted

1 ¼-inch/5mm piece fresh turmeric, grated (or ¼ teaspoon ground)

1 teaspoon cinnamon

1 tablespoon almond butter

Combine all the ingredients with 1 cup/250ml of water in a high-speed blender and blend until smooth. Serve immediately.

Daily Dozen Foods

✗ OTHER FRUITS   ✗ OTHER VEGETABLES   ✗ NUTS AND SEEDS   ✗ BEVERAGES

CHERRY-BERRY SMOOTHIE

MAKES: *1* (2½-CUP/600ML) SERVING • DIFFICULTY: *easy*

This is a great go-to smoothie that can be enjoyed year-round if you keep some berries stashed in the freezer. Mix and match the types of berries (or use other fresh or frozen fruit) to change things up. If your fruit isn't sweet enough, add a soft date or two or a drizzle of Date Syrup (page 3) to taste.

1 cup/100g frozen blueberries

½ cup/110g fresh or frozen pitted cherries

1 frozen ripe banana, cut into chunks before freezing

1 tablespoon ground flaxseeds (or linseeds)

1 tablespoon almond butter

Combine all the ingredients with 1½ cups/360ml of water in a blender and blend until smooth and creamy, about 1 minute. Add more water if you prefer a thinner consistency. Serve immediately.

Daily Dozen Foods

X BERRIES   X OTHER FRUITS   X FLAXSEEDS   X NUTS AND SEEDS   X BEVERAGES

SUPER GREEN SMOOTHIE

MAKES: *1* (2½-CUP/600ML) SERVING • DIFFICULTY: *easy*

You can check off six of the Daily Dozen scorecard boxes with this delicious and refreshing drink. Six with just one smoothie! For a thinner texture, add a little more water, if desired.

2 cups/450g packed fresh baby spinach

1 large apple, cored

1 cup/200g diced pineapple

½ ripe Hass avocado, peeled and pitted

¼ cup/15g packed fresh mint leaves

3 soft Medjool dates, pitted

1 ¼-inch/5mm piece fresh turmeric, grated (or ¼ teaspoon ground)

2 teaspoons blended peeled lemon or lime (see page 3)

1 tablespoon ground flaxseeds (or linseeds)

Ice cubes (optional)

In a blender, combine all the ingredients and blend until completely smooth. Add ⅔ cup/160ml or more of water and ice (if using) and blend until smooth. Serve immediately.

Daily Dozen Foods

X OTHER FRUITS   X GREENS   X OTHER VEGETABLES   X NUTS AND SEEDS   X HERBS AND SPICES   X BEVERAGES

V-12 VEGETABLE BLAST

MAKES: *2* (12-OUNCE/350ML) SERVINGS • DIFFICULTY: *easy*

This is a great way to drink your vegetables!

---

2 cups/450g spinach, red kale or other dark greens

1 or 2 plum tomatoes

1 celery stalk, coarsely chopped

½ red pepper, quartered

1 tablespoon chopped red onion, or 1 small garlic clove

½ jalapeño pepper, seeded (optional, but whoo-hoo!)

2 teaspoons blended peeled lemon (see page 3)

1 apple, cored and quartered

2 teaspoons chlorella (optional)

1 ¼-inch/5mm piece fresh turmeric, grated (or ¼ teaspoon ground)

½ cup ice cubes (about 4 cubes)

Combine all the ingredients with 2 cups/500ml of water in a high-speed blender and blend until smooth. Transfer to large glasses and serve.

Daily Dozen Foods

✗ OTHER FRUITS   ✗ GREENS   ✗ OTHER VEGETABLES   ✗ HERBS AND SPICES   ✗ BEVERAGES

PEOPLE OFTEN ASK ME FOR MORE THAN RECIPES

They want suggestions on how to create meal plans for a week or more. To honor those requests, here are two full weeks of menu preparations. You can also check out my Lighter profile for free meal plans incorporating hundreds of recipes at www.lighter.world/providers/Michael_Greger

WEEK 1

DAY 1

BREAKFAST

Summertime Oatmeal

LUNCH

Curried Chickpea Wraps

V-12 Vegetable Blast

DINNER

Super Salad with Garlic Caesar Dressing
& Hemp Hearts

Courgette Noodles with Avocado-Cashew Alfredo

DESSERT

Strawberry-Banana Nice Cream

DAY 2

BREAKFAST

Burrito Breakfast Bake

LUNCH

Vegetable & Red Bean Gumbo

Cheesy Kale Crisps

DINNER

Miso Soup with Spinach & Dulse

Buckwheat Soba & Edamame
with Almond Butter Sauce

DESSERT

Berry Chocolate Chia Pudding

DAY 3

BREAKFAST

Morning Grain Bowls

LUNCH

Spinach & Mushroom Black Bean Burritos

Edamame Guacamole + raw veggies

DINNER

Mango-Avocado-Kale Salad with
Ginger-Sesame Orange Dressing

Yellow Rice & Black Beans with Broccoli

DESSERT

Fudgy No-Bake Brownies

DAY 4

BREAKFAST

Super Green Smoothie

LUNCH

Black Bean Gazpacho Salad

Pumpkin Seed Dip + raw veggies

DINNER

Stuffed Portobellos with Herbed Mushroom Gravy

Red Cabbage Sauté

DESSERT

Baked Apple Crumbles

DAY 5

BREAKFAST
French Toast with Berry Drizzle
Warm Pear Compote

LUNCH
Kale & White Bean Soup
Three-Seed Crackers

DINNER
Super Salad with Garlic Caesar Dressing
& Hemp Hearts
Roasted Vegetable Lasagna

DESSERT
Very Cherry Nice Cream

DAY 6

BREAKFAST
Frying Pan Sweet Potato Hash
100% whole-grain toast

LUNCH
Beans & Greens Quesadillas
Summer Salsa

DINNER
Portobellos & Greens on Toast
Baked Onion Rings

DESSERT
Two-Berry Pie with Pecan-Sunflower Crust

DAY 7

BREAKFAST
French Toast with Berry Drizzle

LUNCH
Sloppy Jacks

DINNER
Lentil Shepherd's Pie
Roasted Asparagus with Yellow Pepper Béarnaise

DESSERT
Almond-Chocolate Truffles

WEEK 2

DAY 8

BREAKFAST
Summertime Oatmeal

LUNCH
Moroccan Lentil Soup
Cheesy Kale Crisps

DINNER
Garlic Greens Sauté
Mac & Cheese

DESSERT
Raspberry-Peach Crisp

DAY 9

BREAKFAST
Pumpkin Pie Smoothie
Superfood Breakfast Bites

LUNCH
Chopped Vegetable Salad
Champion Vegetable Chilli

DINNER
Quinoa Pilaf with Carrots & Chickpeas
Cauliflower Steaks with Chermoula Sauce

DESSERT
Strawberry-Banana Nice Cream

DAY 10

BREAKFAST
Chocolate Oatmeal

LUNCH
Black Bean Soup with Quinoa & Kale
Beetroot Burgers

DINNER
Pistachio-Spinach Salad with
Strawberry Balsamic Dressing
Whole Wheat Pasta with Lentil Bolognese

DESSERT
Fresh Fruit Skewers with Blackberry Coulis

DAY 11

BREAKFAST
Burrito Breakfast Bake

LUNCH
Smoky Black-Eyed Peas & Spring Greens
Brown rice

DINNER
Chickpea & Cauliflower Curry
Brown rice
Indian-Style Spinach & Tomatoes

DESSERT
Fudgy No-Bake Brownies

DAY 12

BREAKFAST

Superfood Breakfast Bites

Cherry-Berry Smoothie

LUNCH

Veracruz Tempeh Lettuce Wraps

Smoky Roasted Chickpeas

DINNER

Braised Tempeh & Bok Choy
with Spicy Ginger Sauce

Brown rice

DESSERT

No-Bake Oatmeal Walnut Cookies

DAY 13

BREAKFAST

Morning Grain Bowls

LUNCH

Black Bean Burgers

Sesame Red Cabbage & Carrot Slaw

DINNER

Roasted Beetroots with Balsamic-
Braised Beetroot Greens

Stuffed Winter Squash with Black Bean Sauce

DESSERT

Peanut Butter-Banana Nice Cream

DAY 14

BREAKFAST

Frying Pan Sweet Potato Hash

100% whole-grain toast

LUNCH

Kale Salad with Avocado Goddess Dressing

Beans & Greens Quesadillas

DINNER

Lemon-Roasted Brussels Sprouts
& Carrots with Pecans

Red Quinoa Loaf with Golden Gravy

DESSERT

Fresh Fruit Skewers with Blackberry Coulis

KITCHEN TECHNIQUES

Here's a handful of hints and explanations to help you in the kitchen:

BAKING: This dry-heat cooking method takes place in an oven, usually with a temperature below 400°F/200°C, primarily involving foods that lack structure before becoming solid, such as muffins or cakes.

BAKING AND ROASTING WITH SILICONE MATS OR BAKING PARCHMENT: Lining your baking sheets and pans with silicone mats or baking parchment before placing ingredients on them allows you to bake and roast without oil and without the food sticking. It also makes cleanup that much easier.

BRAISING: This cooking method uses both moist and dry heats. Typically, the food is first seared at a high temperature before being finished in a covered pan at a lower temperature with some cooking liquid that may also add flavor. The cooking liquid is then sometimes thickened to create a sauce or gravy.

ROASTING: Similar to baking, this dry-heat cooking method takes place in an oven, usually with a temperature at or above 400°F/200°C. Roasting involves cooking foods that already have a solid structure before the cooking process begins, such as vegetables.

SIMMERING: This is a technique in which foods are cooked in a hot liquid that is kept just below the boiling point of water. To keep a liquid simmering, bring it to a boil and then lower the heat to a point where the bubbles almost stop forming. Simmering is a gentle cooking method often used to cook soup and stews.

SOAKING AND BLENDING NUTS: Some recipes require nuts to be ground into sauces, nut milk or nut cream. Compared with blanched almonds, cashews are softer and will grind more easily into a fine powder. In order to make the smoothest sauce possible, either first grind the nuts into a powder and blend the sauce long enough to achieve a smooth sauce or soak the nuts in water overnight or in hot water for a couple of hours.

STEAMING TEMPEH: Before using tempeh in recipes, it is advisable to steam it over simmering water for 15 to 30 minutes to help mellow its flavor.

STEAMING VEGETABLES: To steam vegetables, bring a few inches of water to a boil in a large saucepan. Arrange the vegetables in a steaming basket and set it over the boiling water, making sure that the vegetables aren't immersed in the water. Cover and let the vegetables steam until they're cooked to the desired tenderness. Check the water level, if needed, to be sure it doesn't all evaporate.

STIR-FRYING: This method of quick cooking over medium-high heat helps maintain the color, flavor and texture of the foods you prepare. When you stir-fry, it's best to have your ingredients prepped and ready to go so they can be quickly tossed into the wok or pan. Different ingredients are added separately to a stir-fry, according to their different cooking times – for example thinly sliced mushrooms stir-fry in a few minutes, whereas diced carrots take longer. Once the ingredients are nearly cooked, add spices or a sauce and stir to coat the ingredients. Although stir-frying in oil is a common method, you can – and should – stir-fry in water instead for a healthier dish without the added empty calories.

WATER-SAUTÉING: This method is a way to sauté ingredients without using oil. To water-sauté, heat 2 tablespoons (or more, depending on the recipe) of water in a frying pan over medium heat. Add your ingredients to the hot liquid and cook, stirring or turning as needed, until the ingredients have softened. In place of water, you can also sauté in wine, vinegar, Vegetable Broth (page 6), and even the liquid from a tin of unsalted beans.

SHOPPING AND STOCKING
THE CUPBOARDS

I wrote this cookbook because people wanted recipes that would help them understand how to apply the principles in *How Not to Die* in their daily diet and to give them handy, delicious ways to get the Daily Dozen and other wonderful Green Light foods into their meals.

That's great if you're already committed to the most healthful way of eating. But I also wrote this book for those of you who may be at the experimental stage, where you are telling yourself, 'Okay, I'm willing to try eating more healthfully, but I'm only going to do it if I like what's on my plate!'

To eat well, it helps to cook well, and to cook well, you need to have the right foods at the ready. And all that starts with shopping.

When I go to the shops, I am thinking mainly about three things: produce, produce and produce. I try to stock the fridge with as many fresh vegetables and fruits as will fit.

A shopping spree in our household means spending almost all of our time in the fresh produce aisle. I love seeing what new items are in season – such as peaches in the summer and squash in the winter. I try to make sure my trolley mimics a rainbow. Besides all shades of greens, I might buy red cabbage, yellow peppers, red apples and blueberries. More colors mean the most plant pigments, which mean more antioxidants.

As part of our produce-gathering mission, I also spend time in the opposite side of the store, the frozen foods section. Sometimes frozen fruits and veggies actually contain more nutrition than fresh ones. Frozen vegetables may be frozen on the day of picking, whereas 'fresh' produce may have been sitting on a ship from the other side of the Earth, losing some of its nutritional value along the way. Local and fresh-picked is best, but not available year-round where I live, which is why I hang out in the frozen foods aisle.

The only times I really fan out into the heart of the store is to buy whole-grain pastas, jarred or Tetra Pak tomato products, tinned beans when I'm not cooking my own, and whole grains, dried beans, nuts and seeds, dried fruit and spices from the bulk aisle. I like to make big batches of beans and greens so I have them always at the ready to instantly improve the nutrition of any dish. I hate to see good food go bad, so it provides that extra motivation to pack in the healthiest of foods.

As well, I keep lots of old bottles and shakers sitting out on the kitchen island. I keep them brimming with spice mixes I've created, chia seeds, pumpkin seeds, dried parsley, dried peppermint, dried dill, ground flaxseeds and dried barberries, all ready to spontaneously add extra texture, flavor and nutrition to meals.

It takes time to build up a truly plant-ter-rific kitchen, and I recommend going at whatever pace you feel comfortable to transition to a fully evidence-based diet. The people who try to adopt a whole-food, plant-based diet cold turkey are often, I'm afraid, the ones who may not keep it up. People who learn to eat well over time, food by food and meal by meal, may do best. They experiment with new foods, delib-erately adding more vegetables to their diet to crowd out some of the less healthy choices and when they can, introducing a new, healthful recipe to their cooking repertoire. Then they find another such recipe, and another, until all of their meals are centered around Green Light foods.

The most important thing to keep in mind is long-term sustainability. It's not what you ate for the first few decades of your life, or even what you eat tomorrow or next week, that matters. It's all about what you eat for the next few decades. So please proceed at whatever pace works best for you. Remember: don't stress if you fall off the wagon from time to time. If you do eat poorly one day, simply try to eat better the next.

Besides these basics, it's also important to find foods you love. And the best way to do that may be to expand your horizons. There are all kinds of exotic beans and greens, so why not select some you aren't as familiar with? How about adzuki beans or gigantes? What about sorrel or kai-lan (Chinese broccoli)? If you're lucky enough to have a large Asian market near you, that's where you can find more unusual produce, such as jackfruit, which looks like a huge, spiky melon with a shredded meatlike tex-ture that can help extend your meatless Monday health streak into taco Tuesday. Although eating healthfully might sound limiting at first, many people tell me that they end up eating a more diverse diet than they ever have before.

Venture into the ethnic sections of your local supermarkets, which span Mexican, Chinese, Indian, Thai, Ethiopian, and beyond. The goal is to find sauces or seasonings that can jazz up the most humble of beans or greens. Most prepared sauces are Yellow or Red Light foods, with added salt, sugar, and fat, but if a not-so-good-for-you sauce dramatically increases your intake of whole plant foods, it may be worth it to use it until you can Google your way to find a Green Light alternative.

Some spice mixes may start out in the Green, such as Italian, jerk, taco, berbere, garam masala and za'atar. Be sure to have some on hand so when you're in the midst of cooking, you can just toss some in the pot without having to worry about the proper ratio of basil-to-oregano (or whatever). That's already been taken care of for you.

To help you stock your kitchen cupboards, the following list is a guide to the foods you may want to have, particularly if you are going to be cooking up the recipes in this book.

CUPBOARDS

artichoke hearts (jarred or frozen)

BEANS: (dried and tinned) black beans, chickpeas, kidney beans, haricot beans, black-eyed peas, pinto beans, lentils, split peas and cannellini beans

chickpea flour

chipotle chillies in adobo

cocoa powder (unsweetened)

curry powder

date sugar

dried chillies

DRIED FRUITS: dates, raisins, apricots, goji berries, figs

dulse seaweed flakes

GRAINS: red, brown or black rice, red or black quinoa, rolled oats

miso paste (white)

mustard (salt free whole-grain)

nut butters and tahini

nutritional yeast (or yeast flakes)

NUTS AND SEEDS: cashews, almonds, pecans, peanuts, walnuts, flaxseeds (or linseeds), sesame seeds, hulled hemp seeds (hemp hearts)

PASTA AND NOODLES: 100% whole-grain or bean-based spaghetti, linguine, fusilli, lasagna, soba

roasted red peppers, jarred

spices and dried herbs

TOMATO PRODUCTS: salt-free jarred, BPA-free tinned or Tetra Pak tomato products (diced, whole, purée, passata, marinara sauce)

TORTILLAS: 100% whole-grain and corn

vanilla pods

vinegars (balsamic, rice, tarragon)

FRESH

FRUITS AND ROOT VEGETABLES: onions, garlic, carrots, sweet potatoes and celery, as well as lemons, limes, bananas, gingerroot and seasonal fruits

LEAFY GREENS: kale, baby spinach, rocket and fresh herbs, as well as crucifers including cauliflower and red cabbage

SALAD INGREDIENTS: lettuce, cucumber, tomato, pepper and avocado, and other vegetables, such as asparagus, green beans, broccoli, mushrooms, squash and corn

tempeh

FROZEN

VEGETABLES: greens, corn kernels, green peas, edamame

FRUIT: blueberries, cherries, strawberries, peaches, mangoes

cooked and portioned rice (black, red or brown), beans and Vegetable Broth (page 6)

ALSO, KEEP ON HAND THE FOLLOWING:

Almond Milk (page 2)

Date Syrup (page 3)

Savory Spice Blend (page 4)

Nutty Parm (page 4)

Umami Sauce (page 5)

Vegetable Broth (page 6)

Healthy Hot Sauce (page 8)

REFERENCES

1. D. Ornish, S. E. Brown, L. W. Scherwitz, et al., 'Can Lifestyle Changes Reverse Coronary Heart Disease? The Lifestyle Heart Trial', *Lancet* 336, no. 8707 (1990): 129–33.

2. J. W. Anderson and K. Ward, 'High-Carbohydrate, High-Fiber Diets for Insulin-Treated Men with Diabetes Mellitus', *Am J Clin Nutr* 32, no. 11 (1979): 2312–21.

3. Kaiser Permanente, 'The Plant-Based Diet: A Healthier Way to Eat', https://share.kaiserpermanente.org/wp-content/uploads/2015/10/The-Plant-Based-Diet-booklet.pdf. 2013, accessed April 10, 2015.

4. T. Monte and I. Pritikin, *Pritikin: The Man Who Healed America's Heart* (Emmaus, PA: Rodale Press; 1988).

5. D. Mozaffarian, E. J. Benjamin, A. S. Go, et al., 'Heart Disease and Stroke Statistics – 2015 Update: A Report from the American Heart Association', *Circulation* 131, no. 4 (2015): e29–322.

6. T. C. Campbell, B. Parpia, and J. Chen, 'Diet, Lifestyle, and the Etiology of Coronary Artery Disease: The Cornell China Study', *Am J Cardiol* 82, no. 10B (1998): 18T–21T.

7. W. A. Thomas, J. N. Davies, R. M. O'Neal, and A. A. Dimakulangan, 'Incidence of Myocardial Infarction Correlated with Venous and Pulmonary Thrombosis and Embolism. A Geographic Study Based on Autopsies in Uganda, East Africa and St. Louis, U.S.A.', *Am J Cardiol* 5 (1960): 41–7.

8. R. D. Voller and W. B. Strong, 'Pediatric Aspects of Atherosclerosis', *Am Heart J* 101, no. 6 (1981): 815–36.

9. C. Napoli, F. P. D'Armiento, FP. Mancini, et al., 'Fatty Streak Formation Occurs in Human Fetal Aortas and Is Greatly Enhanced by Maternal Hypercholesterolemia. Intimal Accumulation of Low Density Lipoprotein and Its Oxidation Precede Monocyte Recruitment into Early Atherosclerotic Lesions', *J Clin Invest* 100, no. 11 (1997): 2680–90.

10. W. F. Enos, R. H. Holmes, and J. Beyer, 'Coronary Disease Among United States Soldiers Killed in Action in Korea: Preliminary Report', *J Am Med Assoc* 152, no. 12 (1953): 1090–93.

11. R. D. Voller and W. B. Strong, 'Pediatric Aspects of Atherosclerosis', *Am Heart J* 101, no. 6 (1981): 815–36.

12. D. Ornish, L. W. Scherwitz, J. H. Billings, et al., 'Intensive Lifestyle Changes for Reversal of Coronary Heart Disease', *JAMA* 280, no. 23 (1998): 2001–7.

13. C. B. Esselstyn Jr, G. Gendy, J. Doyle, M. Golubic, and M. F. Roizen, 'A Way to Reverse CAD?' *J Fam Pract* 63, no. 7 (2014): 356–64b.

14. American Cancer Society, 'Cancer Facts and Figures 2015' (Atlanta: American Cancer Society, 2015); National Heart, Lung, and Blood Institute, NIH, *NHLBI Fact Book, Fiscal Year 2012*, http://www.nhlbi.nih.gov/files/docs/factbook/FactBook2012.pdf, February 2013, accessed March 31, 2015.

15. P. Riso, D. Martini, P. Møller, et al., 'DNA Damage and Repair Activity After Broccoli Intake in Young Healthy Smokers', *Mutagenesis* 25, no. 6 (November 2010): 595–602.

16. I. C. Walda, C. Tabak, H. A. Smit, et al., 'Diet and 20-Year Chronic Obstructive Pulmonary Disease Mortality in Middle-Aged Men from Three European Countries', *Eur J Clin Nutr* 56, no. 7 (2002): 638–43.

17. J. L. Protudjer, G. P. Sevenhuysen, C. D. Ramsey, A. L. Kozyrskyj, and A. B. Becker, 'Low Vegetable Intake Is Associated with Allergic Asthma and Moderate-to-Severe Airway Hyperresponsiveness', *Pediatr Pulmonol* 47, no. 12 (2012): 1159–69.

18. L. G. Wood, M. L. Garg, J. M. Smart, H. A. Scott, D. Barker, and P. G. Gibson, 'Manipulating Antioxidant Intake in Asthma: A Randomized Controlled Trial', *Am J Clin Nutr* 96, no. 3 (2012): 534–43.

19. D. Mozaffarian, E. J. Benjamin, A. S. Go, et al., 'Heart Disease and Stroke Statistics – 2015 Update: A Report from the American Heart Association', *Circulation* 131, no. 4 (2015): e29–322; Centers for Disease Control and Prevention, Deaths: Final Data for 2013 Table 10, 'Number of deaths from 113 selected causes', *National Vital Statistics Report 2016* 64, no. 2.

20. D. E. Threapleton, D. C. Greenwood, C. E. Evans, et al., 'Dietary Fiber Intake and Risk of First Stroke: A Systematic Review and Meta-analysis', *Stroke* 44, no. 5 (2013): 1360–68.

21. L. D'Elia, G. Barba, F. P. Cappuccio, and P. Strazzullo, 'Potassium Intake, Stroke, and Cardiovascular Disease: A Meta-analysis of Prospective Studies', *J Am Coll Cardiol* 57, no. 10 (2011): 1210–19.

22. J. C. de la Torre, 'Alzheimer's Disease Is Incurable but Preventable', *J Alzheimers Dis* 20, no. 3 (2010): 861–70.

23 A. E. Roher, S. L. Tyas, C. L. Maarouf, et al., 'Intracranial Atherosclerosis as a Contributing Factor to Alzheimer's Disease Dementia', *Alzheimers Dement* 7, no. 4 (2011): 436–44; M. Yarchoan, S. X. Xie, M. A. Kling, et al., 'Cerebrovascular Atherosclerosis Correlates with Alzheimer Pathology in Neurodegenerative Dementias', *Brain* 135, part 2 (2012): 3749–56; L. S. Honig, W. Kukull, and R. Mayeux, 'Atherosclerosis and AD: Analysis of Data from the US National Alzheimer's Coordinating Center', *Neurology* 64, no. 3 (2005): 494–500.

24 L. White, H. Petrovitch, G. W. Ross, et al., 'Prevalence of Dementia in Older Japanese-American Men in Hawaii: The Honolulu-Asia Aging Study', *JAMA* 276, no. 12 (1996): 955–60.

25 H. C. Hendrie, A. Ogunniyi, K. S. Hall, et al., 'Incidence of Dementia and Alzheimer Disease in 2 Communities: Yoruba Residing in Ibadan, Nigeria, and African Americans Residing in Indianapolis, Indiana', *JAMA* 285, no. 6 (2001): 739–47.

26 V. Chandra, M. Ganguli, R. Pandav, et al., 'Prevalence of Alzheimer's Disease and Other Dementias in Rural India: The Indo-US Study', *Neurology* 51, no. 4 (1998): 1000–1008.

27 P. S. Shetty, 'Nutrition Transition in India', *Public Health Nutr* 5, no. 1A (2002): 175–82.

28 American Cancer Society, 'Cancer Facts and Figures 2015', Atlanta: American Cancer Society, 2015.

29 T. T. Macdonald and G. Monteleone, 'Immunity, Inflammation, and Allergy in the Gut', *Science* 307, no. 5717 (2005): 1920–25.

30 S. Bengmark, M. D. Mesa, and A. Gill, 'Plant-Derived Health–The Effects of Turmeric and Curcuminoids', *Nutr Hosp* 24, no. 3 (2009): 273–81.

31 A. Hutchins-Wolfbrandt and A. M. Mistry, 'Dietary Turmeric Potentially Reduces the Risk of Cancer', *Asian Pac J Cancer Prev* 12, no. 12 (2011): 3169–73.

32 International Institute for Population Sciences (IIPS) and Macro International. *National Family Health Survey (NFHS-3), 2005-06: India: Volume. 1.* Mumbai: IIPS, 2007. http://dhsprogram.com/pubs/pdf/FRIND3/FRIND3-Vol1andVol2.pdf

33 American Cancer Society, 'Cancer Facts and Figures 2014', Atlanta: American Cancer Society, 2014.

34 A. C. Thiébaut, L. Jiao, D. T. Silverman, et al., 'Dietary Fatty Acids and Pancreatic Cancer in the NIH-AARP Diet and Health Study', *J Natl Cancer Inst* 101, no. 14 (2009): 1001–11.

35 S. Rohrmann, J. Linseisen, U. Nöthlings, et al., 'Meat and Fish Consumption and Risk of Pancreatic Cancer: Results from the European Prospective Investigation into Cancer and Nutrition', *Int J Cancer* 132, no. 3 (2013): 617–24.

36 Centers for Disease Control and Prevention, 'Deaths: Final Data for 2013 Table 10'.

37 A. Gibson, J. Edgar, C. Neville, et al., 'Effect of Fruit and Vegetable Consumption on Immune Function in Older People: A Randomized Controlled Trial', *Am J Clin Nutr* 96, no. 6 (2012): 1429–36.

38 M. Veldhoen, 'Direct Interactions Between Intestinal Immune Cells and the Diet', *Cell Cycle* 11, no. 3 (February 1, 2012): 426–7.

39 L. S. McAnulty, D. C. Nieman, C. L. Dumke, et al., 'Effect of Blueberry Ingestion on Natural Killer Cell Counts, Oxidative Stress, and Inflammation Prior to and after 2.5 H of Running', *Appl Physiol Nutr Metab* 36, no. 6 (2011): 976–84.

40 Centers for Disease Control and Prevention, 'Number (in Millions) of Civilian, Noninstitutionalized Persons with Diagnosed Diabetes, United States, 1980–2011', http://www.cdc.gov/diabetes/statistics/prev/national/figpersons.htm, March 28, 2013, accessed May 3, 2015.

41 Centers for Disease Control and Prevention, 'Deaths: Final Data for 2013 Table 10'.

42 M. Roden, T. B. Price, G. Perseghin, et al., 'Mechanism of Free Fatty Acid-Induced Insulin Resistance in Humans', *J Clin Invest* 97, no. 12 (1996): 2859–65.

43 E. Ginter and V. Simko, 'Type 2 Diabetes Mellitus, Pandemic in 21st Century', *Adv Exp Med Biol* 771 (2012): 42–50.

44 S. Tonstad, T. Butler, R. Yan, and G. E. Fraser, 'Type of Vegetarian Diet, Body Weight, and Prevalence of Type 2 Diabetes', *Diabetes Care* 32, no. 5 (2009): 791–6.

45 R. C. Mollard, B. L. Luhovyy, S. Panahi, M. Nunez, A. Hanley, and G. H. Anderson, 'Regular Consumption of Pulses for 8 Weeks Reduces Metabolic Syndrome Risk Factors in Overweight and Obese Adults', *Br J Nutr* 108, suppl. 1 (2012): S111–22.

46 S. Tonstad, K. Stewart, K. Oda, M. Batech, R. P. Herring, and G. E. Fraser, 'Vegetarian Diets and Incidence of Diabetes in the Adventist Health Study-2', *Nutr Metab Cardiovasc Dis* 23, no. 4 (2013): 292–9.

47 J. W. Anderson and K. Ward, 'High-Carbohydrate, High-Fiber Diets for Insulin-Treated Men with Diabetes Mellitus', *Am J Clin Nutr* 32, no. 11 (1979): 2312–21.

48 S. Bromfield and P. Muntner, 'High Blood Pressure: The Leading Global Burden of Disease Risk Factor and the Need for Worldwide Prevention Programs', *Curr Hypertens Rep* 15, no. 3 (2013): 134–6.

49 S. S. Lim, T. Vos, A. D. Flaxman, et al., 'A Comparative Risk Assessment of Burden of Disease and Injury Attributable to 67 Risk Factors and Risk Factor Clusters in 21 Regions, 1990–2010: A Systematic Analysis for the Global Burden of Disease Study 2010', *Lancet* 380, no. 9859 (2012): 2224–60.

50 D. Mozaffarian, E. J. Benjamin, A. S. Go, et al., 'Heart Disease and Stroke Statistics – 2015 Update: A Report from the American Heart Association', *Circulation* 131, no. 4 (2015): e29–322.

51 T. Nwankwo, S. S. Yoon, V. Burt, and Q. Gu, 'Hypertension among Adults in the United States: National Health and Nutrition Examination Survey, 2011–2012', *NCHS Data Brief* no. 133 (2013): 1–8.

52 C. P. Donnison, 'Blood Pressure in the African Native', *Lancet* 213, no. 5497 (1929): 6–7.

53 M. R. Law, J. K. Morris, and N. J. Wald, 'Use of Blood Pressure Lowering Drugs in the Prevention of Cardiovascular Disease: Meta-analysis of 147 Randomised Trials in the Context of Expectations from Prospective Epidemiological Studies', *BMJ* 338 (2009): b1665.

54 P. Tighe, G. Duthie, N. Vaughan, et al., 'Effect of Increased Consumption of Whole-Grain Foods on Blood Pressure and Other Cardiovascular Risk Markers in Healthy Middle-Aged Persons: A Randomized Controlled Trial', *Am J Clin Nutr* 92, no. 4 (2010): 733–40.

55 D. L. McKay, C. Y. Chen, E. Saltzman, and J. B. Blumberg, '*Hibiscus sabdariffa* L. tea (Tisane) Lowers Blood Pressure in Prehypertensive and Mildly Hypertensive Adults', *J Nutr* 140. no. 2 (2010): 298–303.

56 D. Rodriguez-Leyva, W. Weighell, A. L. Edel, et al., 'Potent Antihypertensive Action of Dietary Flaxseed in Hypertensive Patients', *Hypertension* 62, no. 6 (2013): 1081–9.

57 Centers for Disease Control and Prevention, 'Deaths: Final Data for 2013 Table 10'.

58 E. M. McCarthy and M. E. Rinella, 'The Role of Diet and Nutrient Composition in Nonalcoholic Fatty Liver Disease', *J Acad Nutr Diet* 112, no. 3 (2012): 401–9.

59 J. F. Silverman, W. J. Pories, and J. F. Caro, 'Liver Pathology in Diabetes Mellitus and Morbid Obesity: Clinical, Pathological and Biochemical Considerations', *Pathol Annu* 24 (1989): 275–302.

60 S. Singh, A. M. Allen, Z. Wang, L. J. Prokop, M. H. Murad, and R. Loomba, 'Fibrosis Progression in Nonalcoholic Fatty Liver vs Nonalcoholic Steatohepatitis: A Systematic Review and Meta-analysis of Paired-Biopsy Studies', *Clin Gastroenterol Hepatol* S1542–3565, no. 14 (2014), 00602–8.

61 S. Zelber-Sagi, D. Nitzan-Kaluski, R. Goldsmith, et al., 'Long Term Nutritional Intake and the Risk for Non-alcoholic Fatty Liver Disease (NAFLD): A Population Based Study', *J Hepatol* 47, no. 5 (November 2007): 711–17.

62 Ibid.

63 H. C. Chang, C. N. Huang, D. M. Yeh, S. J. Wang, C. H. Peng, and C. J. Wang, 'Oat Prevents Obesity and Abdominal Fat Distribution, and Improves Liver Function in Humans', *Plant Foods Hum Nutr* 68, no. 1 (2013): 18–23.

64 American Cancer Society, 'Cancer Facts and Figures 2015'.

65 T. J. Key, P. N. Appleby, E. A. Spencer, et al., 'Cancer Incidence in British Vegetarians', *Br J Cancer* 101, no. 1 (2009): 192–7.

66 C. A. Thompson, T. M. Habermann, A. H. Wang, et al., 'Antioxidant Intake from Fruits, Vegetables and Other Sources and Risk of Non-Hodgkin's Lymphoma: The Iowa Women's Health Study', *Int J Cancer* 136, no. 4 (2010): 992–1003.

67 S. G. Holtan, H. M. O'Connor, Z. S. Fredericksen, et al., 'Food-Frequency Questionnaire-Based Estimates of Total Antioxidant Capacity and Risk of Non-Hodgkin Lymphoma', *Int J Cancer* 131, no. 5 (2012;): 1158–68.

68 Centers for Disease Control and Prevention. 'Deaths: Final Data for 2013 Table 10'.

69 J. Coresh, E. Selvin, L. A. Stevens, et al., 'Prevalence of Chronic Kidney Disease in the United States', *JAMA* 298, no. 17 (2007): 2038–47.

70 T. P. Ryan, J. A. Sloand, P. C. Winters, J. P. Corsetti, and S. G. Fisher, 'Chronic Kidney Disease Prevalence and Rate of Diagnosis', *Am J Med* 120, no. 11 (2007): 981–6.

71 J. Lin, F. B. Hu, And G. C. Curhan, 'Associations of Diet with Albuminuria and Kidney Function Decline', *Clin J Am Soc Nephrol* 5, no. 5 (2010): 836–43.

[72] P. Fioretto, R. Trevisan, A. Valerio, et al., 'Impaired Renal Response to a Meat Meal in Insulin-Dependent Diabetes: Role of Glucagon and Prostaglandins', *Am J Physiol* 258, no. 3, part 2 (1990): F675–F83.

[73] A. H. Simon, P. R. Lima, M. Almerinda V. F. Alves, P. V. Bottini, and J. B. Lopes de Faria, 'Renal Haemodynamic Responses to a Chicken or Beef Meal in Normal Individuals', *Nephrol Dial Transplant* 13, no. 9 (1998): 2261–4.

[74] P. Kontessis, S. Jones, R. Dodds, et al., 'Renal, Metabolic and Hormonal Responses to Ingestion of Animal and Vegetable Proteins', *Kidney Int* 38, no. 1 (July 1990): 136–44.

[75] Z. M. Liu, S. C. Ho, Y. M. Chen, N. Tang, and J. Woo, 'Effect of Whole Soy and Purified Isoflavone Daidzein on Renal Function – A 6-Month Randomized Controlled Trial in Equol-Producing Postmenopausal Women with Prehypertension', *Clin Biochem* 47, nos. 13–14 (2014): 1250–56.

[76] American Cancer Society, 'Breast Cancer Facts and Figures 2013–2014', http://www.cancer.org/acs/groups/content/@research/documents/document/acspc-042725.pdf, published 2013, accessed March 10, 2015.

[77] S. E. Steck, M. M. Gaudet, S. M. Eng, et al., 'Cooked Meat and Risk of Breast Cancer – Lifetime versus Recent Dietary Intake', *Epidemiology* 18, no. 3 (2007): 373–82.

[78] C. M. Kitahara, A. Berrington de Gonzhara, N. D. Freedman, et al., 'Total Cholesterol and Cancer Risk in a Large Prospective Study in Korea', *J Clin Oncol* 29, no. 12 (2011): 1592–8.

[79] D. A. Boggs, J. R. Palmer, L. A. Wise, et al., 'Fruit and Vegetable Intake in Relation to Risk of Breast Cancer in the Black Women's Health Study', *Am J Epidemiol* 172, no. 11 (2010): 1268–79.

[80] Q. Li, T. R. Holford, Y. Zhang, et al., 'Dietary Fiber Intake and Risk of Breast Cancer by Menopausal and Estrogen Receptor Status', *Eur J Nutr* 52, no. 1 (2013): 217–23.

[81] Centers for Disease Control and Prevention, 'Deaths: Final Data for 2013, table 18', http://www.cdc.gov/nchs/data/nvsr/nvsr64/nvsr64_02.pdf, accessed March 20, 2015.

[82] N. Sartorius, 'The Economic and Social Burden of Depression', *J Clin Psychiatry*, 62, suppl. 15 (2001): 8–11.

[83] A. C. Tsai, T.-L. Chang, and S.-H. Chi, 'Frequent Consumption of Vegetables Predicts Lower Risk of Depression in Older Taiwanese – Results of a Prospective Population-Based Study', *Public Health Nutr* 15, no. 6 (2012): 1087–92.

[84] F. Gomez-Pinilla and T. T. J. Nguyen, 'Natural Mood Foods: The Actions of Polyphenols against Psychiatric and Cognitive Disorders', *Nutr Neurosci* 15, no. 3 (2012): 127–33.

[85] A. A. Noorbala, S. Akhondzadeh, N. Tahmacebi-Pour, and A. H. Jamshidi, 'Hydro-alcoholic Extract of Crocus sativus L. versus Fluoxetine in the Treatment of Mild to Moderate Depression: A Double-Blind, Randomized Pilot Trial', *J Ethnopharmacol* 97, no. 2 (2005): 281–4.

[86] J. L. Jahn, E. L. Giovannucci, and M. J. Stampfer, 'The High Prevalence of Undiagnosed Prostate Cancer at Autopsy: Implications for Epidemiology and Treatment of Prostate Cancer in the Prostate-Specific Antigen-Era', *Int J Cancer* 137, no. 12 (2015): 2795–2802.

[87] Centers for Disease Control and Prevention, 'Prostate Cancer Statistics', http://www.cdc.gov/cancer/prostate/statistics/index.htm, updated September 2, 2014, accessed March 11, 2015.

[88] D. Ganmaa, X. M. Li, L. Q. Qin, P. Y. Wang, M. Takeda, and A. Sato', 'The Experience of Japan as a Clue to the Etiology of Testicular and Prostatic Cancers', *Med Hypotheses* 60, no. 5 (2003): 724–30.

[89] D. Aune, D. A. Navarro Rosenblatt, D. S. Chan, et al., 'Dairy Products, Calcium, and Prostate Cancer Risk: A Systematic Review and Meta-analysis of Cohort Studies', *Am J Clin Nutr* 101, no. 1 (2015): 87–117.

[90] D. Ornish, G. Weidner, W. R. Fair, et al., 'Intensive Lifestyle Changes May Affect the Progression of Prostate Cancer', *J Urol* 174, no. 3 (2005): 1065–9.

[91] Centers for Disease Control and Prevention, 'Deaths: Final Data for 2013, table 10'.

[92] R. Vogt, D. Bennett, D. Cassady, J. Frost, B. Ritz, and I. Hertz-Picciotto, 'Cancer and Non-cancer Health Effects from Food Contaminant Exposures for Children and Adults in California: A Risk Assessment', *Environ Health* 11 (2012): 83.

[93] European Food Safety Authority, 'Results of the Monitoring of Non Dioxin-like PCBs in Food and Feed', *EFSA Journal* 8, no. 7 (2010): 1701.

[94] H. Arguin, M. Arguin, G. A. Bray, et al., 'Impact of Adopting a Vegan Diet or an Olestra Supplementation on Plasma Organochlorine Concentrations: Results from Two Pilot Studies', *Br J Nutr* 103, no. 10 (2010): 1433–41.

95   J. Lazarou, B. H. Pomeranz, and P. N. Corey, 'Incidence of Adverse Drug Reactions in Hospitalized Patients: A Meta-analysis of Prospective Studies', *JAMA* 279, no. 15 (1998): 1200–1205; B. Starfield, 'Is US Health Really the Best in the World?', *JAMA* 284, no. 4 (2000): 483–5; R. M. Klevens, J. R. Edwards, C. L. Richards, et al., 'Estimating Health Care–Associated Infections and Deaths in U.S. Hospitals, 2002', *Public Health Rep* 122, no. 2 (2007): 160–66; Institute of Medicine, 'To Err Is Human: Building a Safer Health System', http://www.iom.edu/~/media/Files/Report%20Files/1999/To-Err-is-Human/To%20Err%20is%20Human%201999%20%20report%20brief.pdf, November 1999, accessed March 12, 2015.

96   Klevens, Edwards, Richards, et al., 'Estimating Health Care – Associated Infections and Deaths in U.S. Hospitals, 2002'.

97   Lazarou, Pomeranz, and Corey, 'Incidence of Adverse Drug Reactions in Hospitalized Patients'.

98   Institute of Medicine, 'To Err Is Human'.

99   E. Picano, 'Informed Consent and Communication of Risk from Radiological and Nuclear Medicine Examinations: How to Escape from a Communication Inferno', *BMJ* 329, no. 7470 (2004): 849–51.

100   C. W. Schmidt, 'CT Scans: Balancing Health Risks and Medical Benefits', *Environ Health Perspect* 120, no. 3 (2012): A118–21.

101   P. N. Trewby, A. V. Reddy, C. S. Trewby, V. J. Ashton, G. Brennan, and J. Inglis, 'Are Preventive Drugs Preventive Enough? A Study of Patients' Expectation of Benefit from Preventive Drugs', *Clin Med* 2, no. 6 (2002): 527–33.

102   Y. F. Chu, J. Sun, X. Wu, and R. H. Liu, 'Antioxidant and Antiproliferative Activities of Common Vegetables', *J Agric Food Chem* 50, no. 23 (2002): 6910–16.

103   W. Rock, M. Rosenblat, H. Borochov-Neori, N. Volkova, S. Judeinstein, M. Elias, and M. Aviram, 'Effects of Date (Phoenix dactylifera L., Medjool or Hallawi Variety) Consumption by Healthy Subjects on Serum Glucose and Lipid Levels and on Serum Oxidative Status: A Pilot Study', *J Agric Food Chem* 57, no. 17 (September 9, 2009): 8010–17.

104   D. Rodriguez-Leyva, W. Weighell, A. L. Edel, et al., 'Potent Antihypertensive Action of Dietary Flaxseed in Hypertensive Patients', *Hypertension* 62, no. 6 (2013): 1081–9.

105   V. A. Cornelissen, R. Buys, and N. A. Smart, 'Endurance Exercise Beneficially Affects Ambulatory Blood Pressure: A Systematic Review and Meta-analysis', *J Hypertens* 31, no. 4 (2013): 639–48.

106   C. J. Fabian, B. F. Kimler, C. M. Zalles, et al., 'Reduction in Ki-67 in Benign Breast Tissue of High-Risk Women with the Lignan Secoisolariciresinol Diglycoside', *Cancer Prev Res* (Phila) 3, no. 10 (2010): 1342–50.

107   S. Y. Kim, S. Yoon, S. M. Kwon, K. S. Park, and Y. C. Lee-kim, 'Kale Juice Improves Coronary Artery Disease Risk Factors in Hypercholesterolemic Men', *Biomed Environ Sci* 21, no. 2 (2008): 91–7.

108   R. H. Dressendorfer, C. E. Wade, C. Hornick, and G. C. Timmis, 'High-Density Lipoprotein-Cholesterol in Marathon Runners during a 20-Day Road Race', *JAMA* 247, no. 12 (1982): 1715–17.

109   G. K. Hovingh, D. J. Rader, and R. A. Hegele, 'HDL Re-examined', *Curr Opin Lipidol* 26, no. 2 (2015): 127–32.

110   D. B. Haytowitz and S. A. Bhagwat, 'USDA Database for the Oxygen Radical Capacity (ORAC) of Selected Foods, Release 2', Washington, DC: United States Department of Agriculture, 2010.

111   U.S. Department of Agriculture, 'Oxygen Radical Absorbance Capacity (ORAC) of Selected Foods – 2007', http://www.orac-info-portal.de/download/ORAC_R2.pdf, November 2007, accessed April 10, 2015.

112   R. C. Mollard, B. L. Luhovyy, S. Panahi, M. Nunez, A. Hanley, and G. H. Anderson, 'Regular Consumption of Pulses for 8 Weeks Reduces Metabolic Syndrome Risk Factors in Overweight and Obese Adults', *Br J Nutr* 108, suppl. 1 (2012): S111–22.

113   H. C. Hung, K. J. Joshipura, R. Jiang, et al., 'Fruit and Vegetable Intake and Risk of Major Chronic Disease', *J Natl Cancer Inst* 96, no. 21 (2004): 1577–84.

114   K. J. Joshipura, F. B. Hu, J. E. Manson, et al., 'The Effect of Fruit and Vegetable Intake on Risk for Coronary Heart Disease', *Ann Intern Med* 134, no. 12 (2001): 1106–14.

115   K. J. Joshipura, A. Ascherio, J. E. Manson, et al., 'Fruit and Vegetable Intake in Relation to Risk of Ischemic Stroke', *JAMA* 282, no. 13 (1999): 1233–9.

116   Y. F. Chu, J. Sun, X. Wu, and R. H. Liu, 'Antioxidant and Antiproliferative Activities of Common Vegetables', *J Agric Food Chem* 50, no. 23 (2002): 6910–16.

117   M. N. Chen, C. C. Lin, and C. F. Liu, 'Efficacy of Phytoestrogens for Menopausal Symptoms: A Meta-analysis and Systematic Review', *Climacteric* 18, no. 2 (2015): 260–69.

118   C. Nagata, T. Mizoue, K. Tanaka, et al., 'Soy Intake and Breast Cancer Risk: An Evaluation Based on a Systematic Review of Epidemiologic Evidence among the Japanese Population', *Jpn J Clin Oncol* 44, no. 3 (2014): 282–95.

119 F. Chi, R. Wu, Y. C. Zeng, R. Xing, Y. Liu, and Z. G. Xu, 'Post-diagnosis Soy Food Intake and Breast Cancer Survival: A Meta-analysis of Cohort Studies', *Asian Pac J Cancer Prev* 14, no. 4 (2013): 2407–12.

120 E. L. Richman, P. R. Carroll, and J. M. Chan, 'Vegetable and Fruit Intake after Diagnosis and Risk of Prostate Cancer Progression', *Int J Cancer* 131, no. 1 (2012): 201–10.

121 S. S. Nielsen, G. M. Franklin, W. T. Longstreth, P. D. Swanson, and H. Checkoway, 'Nicotine from Edible Solanaceae and Risk of Parkinson Disease', *Ann Neurol* 74, no. 3 (2013): 472–7.

122 Y. F. Chu, J. Sun, X. Wu, and R. H. Liu, 'Antioxidant and Antiproliferative Activities of Common Vegetables', *J Agric Food Chem* 50, no. 23 (2002). 6910–16.

123 S. C. Jeong, S. R. Koyyalamudi, and G. Pang, 'Dietary Intake of Agaricusbisporus White Button Mushroom Accelerates Salivary Immunoglobulin A Secretion in Healthy Volunteers', *Nutrition* 28, no. 5 (2012): 527–31.

124 M. Jesenak, M. Hrubisko, J. Majtan, Z. Rennerova, and P. Banovcin, 'Anti-allergic Effect of Pleuran (β-glucan from Pleurotus ostreatus) in Children with Recurrent Respiratory Tract Infections', *Phyto-ther Res* 28, no. 3 (2014): 471–4.

125 M. Maghbooli, F. Golipour, A. Moghimi Esfandabadi, and M. Yousefi, 'Comparison between the Efficacy of Ginger and Sumatriptan in the Ablative Treatment of the Common Migraine', *Phytother Res* 28, no. 3 (2014): 412–15.

126 F. Kashefi, M. Khajehei, M. Tabatabaeichehr, M. Alavinia, and J. Asili, 'Comparison of the Effect of Ginger and Zinc Sulfate on Primary Dysmenorrhea: A Placebo-Controlled Randomized Trial', *Pain Manag Nurs* 15, no. 4 (2014): 826–33.

127 World Cancer Research Fund/American Institute for Cancer Research, 'Food, Nutrition, Physical Activity, and the Prevention of Cancer: A Global Perspective', Washington, DC: AICR, 2007.

128 G. E. Fraser and D. J. Shavlik, 'Ten Years of Life: Is It a Matter of Choice?' *Arch Intern Med* 181, no. 13 (2001): 1645–52.

129 N. Annema, J. S. Heyworth, S. A. Mcnaughton, B. Iacopetta, and L. Fritschi, 'Fruit and Vegetable Consumption and the Risk of Proximal Colon, Distal Colon, and Rectal Cancers in a Case-Control Study in Western Australia', *J Am Diet Assoc* 111, no. 10 (2011): 1479–90.

130 Y. F. Chu, J. Sun, X. Wu, and R. H. Liu, 'Antioxidant and Antiproliferative Activities of Common Vegetables', *J Agric Food Chem* 50, no. 23 (2002): 6910–16.

131 M. Murphy, K. Eliot, R. M. Heuertz, and E. Weiss, 'Whole Beetroot Consumption Acutely Improves Running Performance', *J Acad Nutr Diet* 111, no. 4 (2012): 548–52.

132 V. Kapil, R. S. Khambata, A. Robertson, M. J. Caulfield, and A. Ahluwalia, 'Dietary Nitrate Provides Sustained Blood Pressure Lowering in Hypertensive Patients: A Randomized, Phase 2, Double-Blind, Placebo-Controlled Study', *Hypertension* 65, no. 2 (2015): 320–27.

133 M. Cruz-Correa, D. A. Shoskes, P. Sanchez, et al., 'Combination Treatment with Curcumin and Quercetin of Adenomas in Familial Adenomatous Polyposis', *Clin Gastroenterol Hepatol* 4, no. 8 (2006): 1035–8.

134 C. Galeone, C. Pelucchi, R. Talamini, et al., 'Onion and Garlic Intake and the Odds of Benign Prostatic Hyperplasia', *Urology* 70, no. 4 (2007): 672–6.

135 S. Gallus, R. Talamini, A. Giacosa, et al., 'Does an Apple a Day Keep the Oncologist Away?' *Ann Oncol* 16, no. 11 (2005): 1841–4.

INDEX

Page numbers in italic indicate photographs.

Advanced glycation end products (AGEs), 108
Africa, xiv, 9, 118, 124
African American women, xviii
AGEs. *See* Advanced glycation end products
Almonds
    almond butter, 2
    Almond Butter Sauce, 146
    Almond Milk, xi, 2, 7, 12, 16, 22, 111, 121, 130,
        180, 200, 209
    Almond-Chocolate Truffles, *186*, 187
Alzheimer's disease, xiii–xiv
Antidepressants, xviii
Antioxidants, xvii, 8, 30, 56, 59, 76, 106, 108, 227
Appetizers, 28–9
    Artichoke-Spinach Dip, 30, *31*
    Black-Eyed Peas & Roasted Red Pepper Dip, 36, *37*
    Cheesy Kale Crisps, 42, *43*
    Edamame Guacamole, 38, *39*
    Lemony Hummus, *32*, 33
    Pumpkin Seed Dip, 35
    Smoky Roasted Chickpeas, 44, *45*
    Summer Salsa, *40*, 41
    Three-Seed Crackers, 34
Apples
    Baked Apple Crumbles, 190, *191*
    benefits from, 190
Arrabiata, 108, *109*
Arthritis, 70
Artichoke-Spinach Dip, 30, *31*
Asparagus, 164, *165*

Asthma, xiii
Atherosclerotic plaque buildup, xiv
Avocado
    Avocado Goddess Dressing, 72, *73*
    Avocado-Cashew Alfredo, *104*, 105
    Edamame Guacamole, 38, *39*
    Mango-Avocado-Kale Salad with Ginger-Sesame
        Orange Dressing, 80, *81*

B vitamins, x
Bacteria, xv
Bahri dates, 8
Baked Apple Crumbles, 190, *191*
Baked Onion Rings, 180, *181*
Baking parchment, 225
Balsamic-Braised Beetroot Greens, 168
Balsamic-Date Glaze, 8, 176, *177*
Bananas
    Banana-Chocolate Smoothie, 210, *211*
    Strawberry-Banana Nice Cream, *196*, 197
Beans, 122–3. *See also* Soyabean foods
    Bean Patties with Harissa, 138, *139*
    Beans & Greens Quesadillas, *100*, 101
    benefits from, 138
    Black Bean Burgers, 88, *89*
    Black Bean Gazpacho Salad, 74, 75
    Black Bean Sauce, *154*, 155
    Black Bean Soup with Quinoa & Kale, 56, *57*
    Black-Eyed Peas & Roasted Red Pepper Dip, 36, *37*
    cancer and, 138
    Chickpea & Vegetable Tagine, 124, *125*
    cooking tips for, 2

Curried Chickpea Wraps, 92, *93*
Edamame Guacamole, 38, *39*
Frying Pan Sweet Potato Hash, *26*, 27
Kale & White Bean Soup, 48, *49*
Lemony Hummus, *32*, 33
Lentil Bolognese, 150, *151*
Lentil Shepherd's Pie, *132*, 133
Louisiana Soy Curls, *136*, 137
Moroccan Lentil Soup, 63
Pesto Carrot Noodles with White Beans &
    Tomatoes, 106, *107*
Quinoa Pilaf with Carrots & Chickpeas, *148*, 149
shopping for, 229
Smoky Black-Eyed Peas & Spring Greens, *126*, 127
Spinach & Mushroom Black Bean Burritos, 94, *95*
Summer Garden Gazpacho, 60, *61*
Three-Bean Chilli, 64, *65*
Vegetable & Red Bean Gumbo, 54, *55*
Yellow Rice & Black Beans with Broccoli, 152, *153*
Yellow Split Pea Dal with Watercress, 134, *135*
Beetroots
Beetroot Burgers, 98, *99*
benefits from, 169
for high blood pressure, 169
Roasted Beetroots with Balsamic-Braised Beetroot
    Greens, 168
Beriberi, x
Berries
Berry Chocolate Chia Pudding, 200, *201*
Berry Drizzle, 16, *17*
Blackberry Coulis, 192, *193*
blueberries, xv
Cherry-Berry Smoothie, *214*, 215
Raspberry-Peach Crisp, *194*, 195
Strawberry Balsamic Dressing, 84, *85*
Strawberry-Banana Nice Cream, *196*, 197
Two-Berry Pie with Pecan-Sunflower Crust, *202*,
    203
Beverages, 204–5. *See also* Smoothies
Golden Chai, *208*, 209
Lemon-Ginger Cooler, 206, *207*
water, 206
Bisphenol A (BPA), 33

Black beans
Black Bean Burgers, 88, *89*
Black Bean Gazpacho Salad, *74*, 75
Black Bean Sauce, *154*, 155
Black Bean Soup with Quinoa & Kale, 56, *57*
Spinach & Mushroom Black Bean Burritos, 94, *95*
Yellow Rice & Black Beans with Broccoli, 152, *153*
Black Women's Health Study, xviii
Blackberry Coulis, 192, *193*
Black-eyed peas
Black-Eyed Peas & Roasted Red Pepper Dip, 36, *37*
Smoky Black-Eyed Peas & Spring Greens, *126*, 127
Blood cancers, xvii
Blood cells, xv
Blueberries, xv
Body mass index (BMI), xv
Bok choy, 128, *129*
BPA. *See* Bisphenol A
Brain diseases
Alzheimer's disease, xiii–xiv
high blood pressure and, xvi
stroke, xiii–xiv, xvi
whole-food, plant-based nutrition for, xiii xiv
Braised Tempeh & Bok Choy with Spicy Ginger Sauce,
    128, *129*
Braising, 225
Breakfast, 10–11
Burrito Breakfast Bake, 24, *25*
Chocolate Oatmeal, *20*, 21
French Toast with Berry Drizzle, 16, *17*
Frying Pan Sweet Potato Hash, *26*, 27
Morning Grain Bowls, 22, *23*
Summertime Oatmeal, 12, *13*
Superfood Breakfast Bites, *14*, 15
Warm Pear Compote, 18, *19*
Breast cancer
in African American women, xviii
cholesterol and, xvii–xviii
flaxseeds for, 15
garlic for, 7
soyabean foods and, 98
whole-food, plant-based nutrition for, xvii–xviii
Broccoli

for cancer prevention, xvii
for infections, preventing, xv
lung diseases and, xiii
Yellow Rice & Black Beans with Broccoli, 152, *153*
Broth, 6
Brown rice, x
Brownies, 198, *199*
Brussels sprouts, *166*, 167
Buckwheat Soba & Edamame with Almond Butter
      Sauce, 146
Buffalo Cauliflower, 7, 183
Burgers
      Beetroot Burgers, 98, *99*
      Black Bean Burgers, 88, *89*
Burritos
      Burrito Breakfast Bake, 24, *25*
      Spinach & Mushroom Black Bean Burritos, 94, *95*

C

Cabbage
      benefits from, 76
      Red Cabbage Saute, *172*, *173*
      Sesame Red Cabbage & Carrot Slaw, 76, 77
Campbell, Emeritus T. Colin, xii–xiii
Cancer
      blood, xvii
      breast, xvii–xviii, 7, 15, 98
      colon, xiv, 167
      digestive, xiv–xv, 7, 180
      EPIC study on, xv
      grilled or smoked meat and, xvii
      lung, xiii
      National Institutes of Health-AARP study on, xiv
            –xv
      pancreatic cancer, xiv–xv, 7
      prostate cancer, xviii, 7
      rectal, xiv
      stomach, 7
Cancer-fighting foods
      beans as, 138
      broccoli as, xvii

Brussels sprouts as, 167
cauliflower as, 115
curry powder as, xiv
flaxseeds as, 15
garlic as, 7
onions as, 180
phytates, xiv
soyabean foods as, 98
spinach as, 95
turmeric as, xiv
Cardamom, 63
Carrageenan, 2
Carrots
      Lemon-Roasted Brussels Sprouts & Carrots with
            Pecans, *166*, 167
      Pesto Carrot Noodles with White Beans &
            Tomatoes, 106, *107*
      Quinoa Pilaf with Carrots & Chickpeas, *148*, 149
      Sesame Red Cabbage & Carrot Slaw, 76, 77
Cashews, *104*, 105
Cauliflower
      Buffalo Cauliflower, 7, 183
      cancer and, 115
      Cauliflower Mash, *174*, 175
      Cauliflower Steaks with Chermoula Sauce, 118, *119*
      Chickpea & Cauliflower Curry, 130, *131*
      Curried Cauliflower Soup, *58*, 59
      Frying Pan Sweet Potato Hash, 26, 27
      Whole Roasted Cauliflower with Lemon Tahini
            Sauce, *114*, 115
Center for Alzheimer's Research, xiv
Ceylon cinnamon, 63
Chai, *208*, 209
Champion Vegetable Chilli, 66, 67
Cheesy Kale Crisps, 42, *43*
Chermoula Sauce, 118, *119*
Cherry-Berry Smoothie, *214*, 215
Chicken
      digestive cancers and, xv
      liver disease and, xvi
      toxic heavy metals in, xix

Chickpeas
    benefits from, 92
    Chickpea & Cauliflower Curry, 130, *131*
    Chickpea & Vegetable Tagine, 124, *125*
    Curried Chickpea Wraps, 92, *93*
    Lemony Hummus, *32*, 33
    Quinoa Pilaf with Carrots & Chickpeas, *148*, 149
    Smoky Roasted Chickpeas, 44, *45*
Chilli
    Champion Vegetable Chilli, 66, *67*
    Three-Bean Chilli, 64, *65*
    variations of, 64
The China Study (Campbell), xii–xiii
China-Cornell-Oxford Project, xii–xiii
Chocolate
    Almond-Chocolate Truffles, *186*, 187
    Banana-Chocolate Smoothie, 210, *211*
    Berry Chocolate Chia Pudding, 200, *201*
    Chocolate Oatmeal, *20*, 21
    Fudgy No-Bake Brownies, 198, *199*
Cholesterol
    breast cancer and, xvii–xviii
    in coronary heart disease, xiii
    high, xiii
    kale and, 56
    kidney disease and, xvii
Chopped Vegetable Salad, 78, *79*
Chronic obstructive pulmonary disease (COPD), xiii
Cinnamon, 63
Cirrhosis, xvi
Colon cancer, xiv, 167
Cookies, *188*, 189
Cooking methods, 225–6
Cooking tips, 2–3
COPD. *See* Chronic obstructive pulmonary disease
Coronary heart disease, x
    Campbell on, xii–xiii
    cholesterol in, xiii
    Esselstyn on, xiii
    Ornish on, xiii
    whole-food, plant-based nutrition for, xi, xii–xiii
Courgettes, *104*, 105
Crohn's disease, 4
Culinary exploration, 30, 55

Culinary variety, 55
Curry powder
    as cancer-fighting food, xiv
    Chickpea & Cauliflower Curry, 130, *131*
    Curried Cauliflower Soup, *58*, 59
    Curried Chickpea Wraps, 92, *93*

D

Daily Dozen, xx–xxi. *See also specific recipes*
Dal, 134, *135*
Dates
    Bahri, 8
    Balsamic-Date Glaze, 8, 176, *177*
    date sugar, 3
    Date Syrup, 3, 5, 12, 16, 21, 22, *23*, 44, 70, 72, 76,
        80, 84, 190, 200, 209, 210, 215
    dried, 8
Depression, xviii
Desserts and sweets, 184–5
    Almond-Chocolate Truffles, *186*, 187
    Baked Apple Crumbles, 190, *191*
    Berry Chocolate Chia Pudding, 200, *201*
    Fresh Fruit Skewers with Blackberry Coulis, 192,
        193
    Fudgy No-Bake Brownies, 198, *199*
    No-Bake Oatmeal Walnut Cookies, *188*, 189
    Raspberry-Peach Crisp, *194*, 195
    Strawberry-Banana Nice Cream, *196*, 197
    Two-Berry Pie with Pecan-Sunflower Crust, *202*,
        203
Diabetes. *See* Type 2 diabetes
Diet
    disease and, viii–xi
    healthiest, x
    on holidays and special occasions, xi
Digestive cancers
    chicken and, xv
    onions and, 180
    stomach cancer, 7
    whole-food, plant-based nutrition for, xiv–xv
Dips and spreads
    Artichoke-Spinach Dip, 30, *31*

Black-Eyed Peas & Roasted Red Pepper Dip, 36, *37*
Edamame Guacamole, 38, *39*
Lemony Hummus, *32*, 33
Pumpkin Seed Dip, 35
Summer Salsa, *40*, 41
Diseases. *See also specific diseases*
diet and, viii–xi
spinach for, 95
turmeric for, 70
whole-food, plant-based nutrition and, xi
in womb, xiii
Doctors and medical care, viii–x, xix
Double-batch recipes, 2
Dressings. *See* Salads and dressings
Dried dates, 8
Dulse, 51

E

Edamame
Buckwheat Soba & Edamame with Almond Butter
Sauce, 146
Edamame Guacamole, *38*, *39*
Emphysema, xiii
EPIC study. *See* European Prospective Investigation into
Cancer and Nutrition study
Esselstyn, Caldwell, Jr., xiii
European Prospective Investigation into Cancer and
Nutrition (EPIC) study, xv

F

Fiber, xiv
Financial savings, ix
Flaxseeds
for breast cancer, 15
for high blood pressure, 15
ways to use, 34
Food packaging, 33
Fortified refined grains, x
French toast

French Toast with Berry Drizzle, 16, *17*
Warm Pear Compote for, 18, *19*
Fresh Fruit Skewers with Blackberry Coulis, 192, *193*
Frozen foods, 227, 229
Fruit. *See also specific fruit*
Fresh Fruit Skewers with Blackberry Coulis, 192,
193
shopping for, 229
as snack, 41
Frying Pan Sweet Potato Hash, *26*, 27
Fudgy No-Bake Brownies, 198, *199*

G

Garlic
for cancer prevention, 7
Garlic Caesar Dressing, *82*, 83
Garlic Greens Sauté, 178
Roasted Garlic, 6
Gazpacho
Black Bean Gazpacho Salad, 74, 75
Summer Garden Gazpacho, 60, *61*
Ginger
benefits from, 128
Ginger-Sesame Orange Dressing, 80, *81*
Lemon-Ginger Cooler, 206, *207*
Spicy Ginger Sauce, 128, *129*
Golden Chai, *208*, *209*
Golden Gravy, 156–7, *157*
Golden Quinoa Tabbouleh, 70, *71*
Grains, 140–41
Black Bean Soup with Quinoa & Kale, 56, *57*
brown rice, x
Buckwheat Soba & Edamame with Almond Butter
Sauce, 146
Chickpea & Vegetable Tagine, 124, *125*
cooking tips for, 2
fortified, x
Golden Quinoa Tabbouleh, 70, *71*
Hoppin' John Stuffed Spring Greens Rolls, 158, *159*
Mac & Cheese, *142*, 143
Morning Grain Bowls, 22, *23*
Quinoa Pilaf with Carrots & Chickpeas, *148*, 149

Red Quinoa Loaf with Golden Gravy, 156–7, *157*

refined, x

Roasted Vegetable Lasagna, *110*, 111

shopping for, 229

Rocket Pesto Pasta with Roasted Vegetables, *160*, 161

Stuffed Winter Squash with Black Bean Sauce, *154*, 155

teff, 98

Vegetable Unfried Rice, 144, *145*

wheat, x

white rice, x

Whole Wheat Pasta with Lentil Bolognese, 150, *151*

Yellow Rice & Black Beans with Broccoli, 152, *153*

Green Light foods, xi, 2

Greens. *See also specific greens*

Balsamic-Braised Beetroot Greens, 168

Beans & Greens Quesadillas, *100*, 101

Garlic Greens Sauté, 178

Portobellos & Greens on Toast, 121

shopping for, 229

Super Green Smoothie, 216, *217*

ten ways to eat, 178

Guacamole, 38, *39*

Gumbo, 54, *55*

H

Harissa, 9, 138, *139*

Harvard University, xvii

Health

Black Women's Health Study, xviii

Iowa Women's Health Study, xvii

power over, viii–ix

Healthiest diet, x

Healthy Hot Sauce, 8, 27, 52, 94, 127, 137, 158, 183

Heart disease. *See* Coronary heart disease

Heavy metals, xix

Hemp hearts, *82*, 83

Herbed Mushroom Gravy, 112, *113*

Hidradenitis suppurativa, 4

High blood pressure

beetroot for, 169

brain diseases and, xvi

flaxseeds for, 15

whole-food, plant-based nutrition for, xvi

High cholesterol, xiii

Holidays and special occasions, xi

Hoppin' John Stuffed Spring Greens Rolls, 158, *159*

Hot sauce, 8

How Not to Die (Greger), viii–xi

synopsis of, xii–xix

Hyperfiltration, of kidneys, xvii

Hypertension. *See* High blood pressure

I

Ice cream, *196*, 197

Ikeda, Kikunae, 5

Immune function, 121

Indian-Style Spinach and Tomatoes, 170, *171*

Infections, preventing, xv

Inflammation, xvii

Inflammatory conditions, 4, 70

Influenza, xv

Insulin, xv

Intraepithelial lymphocytes, xv

Iodine, 51

Iowa Women's Health Study, xvii

J

Jackfruit, *90*, 91

K

Kale

benefits from, 56

Black Bean Soup with Quinoa & Kale, 56, *57*

Cheesy Kale Crisps, 42, *43*

cholesterol and, 56

Ginger-Sesame Orange Dressing, 80, *81*
Kale Salad with Avocado Goddess Dressing, 72, *73*
Kale & White Bean Soup, 48, *49*
Mango-Avocado-Kale Salad with Ginger-Sesame
    Orange Dressing, 80, *81*
Kidney disease, xv, xvii
Kitchen techniques, 225–6
Kombu, 51

Lasagna, *110*, 111
Lead, xix
Legumes. *See* Beans
Lemons
    lemon juice, 3
    Lemon Tahini Sauce, *114*, 115
    Lemon-Ginger Cooler, 206, *207*
    Lemon-Roasted Brussels Sprouts & Carrots with
        Pecans, *166*, 167
    Lemony Hummus, *32*, 33
Lentils
    Lentil Bolognese, 150, *151*
    Lentil Shepherd's Pie, *132*, 133
    Moroccan Lentil Soup, 63
Lettuce, *96*, 97. *See also* Salads and Dressings
Leukemia, xvii
Lime juice, 3
Liver disease, xvi
Louisiana Soy Curls, *136*, 137
Lung cancer, xiii
Lung diseases, xiii
Lymphoma, xvii

M

Mac & Cheese, *142*, 143
Main dishes, 102–3
    Bean Patties with Harissa, 138, *139*
    Braised Tempeh & Bok Choy with Spicy Ginger
        Sauce, 128, *129*
    Buckwheat Soba & Edamame with Almond Butter
        Sauce, 146
    Cauliflower Steaks with Chermoula Sauce, 118, *119*
    Chickpea & Cauliflower Curry, 130, *131*
    Chickpea & Vegetable Tagine, 124, *125*
    Courgette Noodles with Avocado-Cashew Alfredo,
        104, 105
    Hoppin' John Stuffed Spring Greens Rolls, 158, *159*
    Lentil Shepherd's Pie, *132*, 133
    Louisiana Soy Curls, *136*, 137
    Mac & Cheese, *142*, 143
    Pesto Carrot Noodles with White Beans &
        Tomatoes, 106, *107*
    Portobellos & Greens on Toast, 121
    Quinoa Pilaf with Carrots & Chickpeas, *148*, 149
    Red Quinoa Loaf with Golden Gravy, 156–7, *157*
    Roasted Vegetable Lasagna, *110*, 111
    Rocket Pesto Pasta with Roasted Vegetables, *160*,
        161
    Smoky Black-Eyed Peas & Spring Greens, *126*, 127
    Spaghetti Squash Arrabiata, 108, *109*
    Stuffed Portobellos with Herbed Mushroom Gravy,
        112, *113*
    Stuffed Winter Squash with Black Bean Sauce, *154*,
        155
    Vegetable Stacks with Tomato-Red Pepper Coulis,
        116, *117*
    Vegetable Unfried Rice, 144, *145*
    Whole Roasted Cauliflower with Lemon Tahini
        Sauce, *114*, 115
    Whole Wheat Pasta with Lentil Bolognese, 150, *151*
    Yellow Rice & Black Beans with Broccoli, 152, *153*
    Yellow Split Pea Dal with Watercress, 134, *135*
Mainstream medicine, viii–x, xii
Mango, 80, *81*
Medical radiation, xix
Medications, viii–x, xvi
Menstrual cramps, 128
Mercury, xix
Miso, 7
    Miso Soup with Spinach & Dulse, 51
Morning Grain Bowls, 22, *23*
Moroccan Lentil Soup, 63
Multiple myeloma, xvii
Mushrooms
    benefits from, 113, 121
    Portobellos & Greens on Toast, 121
    Spinach & Mushroom Black Bean Burritos, 94, *95*

Stuffed Portobellos with Herbed Mushroom Gravy, 112, *113*

N

NAFLD. *See* Nonalcoholic fatty liver disease
National Institutes of Health-AARP study, xiv–xv
Natural killer cells, xv
No-Bake Oatmeal Walnut Cookies, *188*, 189
Nonalcoholic fatty liver disease (NAFLD), xvi
Nutrition. *See* Diet; Whole-food, plant-based nutrition
Nutritional yeast, 4, 44
NutritionFacts.org, viii, xii
Nuts and seeds
    almond butter, 2
    Almond Butter Sauce, 146
    Almond Milk, xi, 2
    Almond-Chocolate Truffles, *186*, 187
    benefits from, 108, 146
    cashews, *104*, 105
    cooking, 108
    flaxseeds, 15, 34
    Nutty Parm, 4, 105, 106, 108, 111, 150, 161
    pecans, *166*, 167, *202*, 203
    Pistachio-Spinach Salad with Strawberry Balsamic Dressing, 84, *85*
    Pumpkin Seed Dip, 35
    raw, 108
    Sesame Red Cabbage & Carrot Slaw, 76, *77*
    shopping for, 229
    soaking and blending, 225
    Three-Seed Crackers, 34
    walnuts, 106, *188*, 189

O

Oatmeal, xi
    Chocolate Oatmeal, *20*, 21
    No-Bake Oatmeal Walnut Cookies, *188*, 189
    Summertime Oatmeal, 12, *13*
    Warm Pear Compote for, 18, *19*

Oats, x
Okra, 54, *55*
Onions, 180, *181*
Oranges, 80, *81*
Ornish, Dean, x, xiii, xviii

P

Pancreatic cancer, xiv–xv, 7
Paprika, 63
Parkinson's disease
    peppers for, 117
    whole-food, plant-based nutrition for, xix
Pasta
    Buckwheat Soba & Edamame with Almond Butter Sauce, 146
    Mac & Cheese, *142*, 143
    Roasted Vegetable Lasagna, *110*, 111
    Rocket Pesto Pasta with Roasted Vegetables, *160*, 161
    shopping for, 229
    Whole Wheat Pasta with Lentil Bolognese, 150, *151*
Papaya, 80
PCB. *See* Polychlorinated biphenyl
Peaches, *194*, 195
Pears, 18, *19*
Peas, 176
Pecans
    Lemon-Roasted Brussels Sprouts & Carrots with Pecans, *166*, 167
    Two-Berry Pie with Pecan-Sunflower Crust, *202*, 203
Peppers
    benefits from, 117
    Black-Eyed Peas & Roasted Red Pepper Dip, 36, *37*
    Harissa, 9
    Healthy Hot Sauce, 8
    for Parkinson's disease, 117
    roasting, 9
    Summer Salsa, *40*, 41
    Tomato-Red Pepper Coulis, 116, *117*
    Yellow Pepper Béarnaise, 164, *165*
Permanente, Kaiser, xi

Pesto
    Pesto Carrot Noodles with White Beans &
        Tomatoes, 106, *107*
    Rocket Pesto Pasta with Roasted Vegetables, *160*,
        161
Phytates, xiv
Pie
    Pumpkin Pie Smoothie, 212, *213*
    Two-Berry Pie with Pecan-Sunflower Crust, *202*,
        203
Pistachio-Spinach Salad with Strawberry Balsamic
        Dressing, 84, *85*
Plant pigments, 56, 59, 227
The Plant-Based Diet: A Healthier Way to Eat
        (Permanente), xi
Pneumonia, xv
Polychlorinated biphenyl (PCB), xix
Polyps, 70
Popcorn, 44
Portobellos & Greens on Toast, 121
Potassium, xiv
Pregnancy, xiii
Prepping tips, 2
Pritikin, Nathan, xi, xii
Processed foods, x, xi
Prostate cancer, xviii, 7
Pudding, 200, *201*
Pumpkin Pie Smoothie, 212, *213*
Pumpkin Seed Dip, 35

Q

Quesadillas, *100*, 101
Quinoa
    Black Bean Soup with Quinoa & Kale, 56, *57*
    Chickpea & Vegetable Tagine, 124, *125*
    Golden Quinoa Tabbouleh, 70, *71*
    Quinoa Pilaf with Carrots & Chickpeas, *148*, 149
    Red Quinoa Loaf with Golden Gravy, 156–7, *157*

R

Ranch Dressing, 7, 183
Raspberry-Peach Crisp, *194*, 195
Raw nuts and seeds, 108
Rectal cancer, xiv
Red beans, 54, *55*
Red Cabbage Sauté, *172*, 173
Red Light foods, xi, 2
Red Quinoa Loaf with Golden Gravy, 156–7, *157*
Refined grains, x
Rice
    brown, x
    Vegetable Unfried Rice, 144, *145*
    white, x
    Yellow Rice & Black Beans with Broccoli, 152, *153*
Roasted Asparagus with Yellow Pepper Béarnaise, 164,
        165
Roasted Beetroots with Balsamic-Braised Beetroot
        Greens, 168
Roasted Garlic, 6, 7, 35
Roasted Vegetable Lasagna, *110*, 111
Roasting, 9, 225
Rocket Pesto Pasta with Roasted Vegetables, *160*, 161

S

Saffron, xviii
Salads and dressings, 68–9
    Black Bean Gazpacho Salad, 74, *75*
    Chopped Vegetable Salad, *78*, 79
    Golden Quinoa Tabbouleh, 70, *71*
    Kale Salad with Avocado Goddess Dressing, 72, *73*
    Mango-Avocado-Kale Salad with Ginger-Sesame
        Orange Dressing, 80, *81*
    Pistachio-Spinach Salad with Strawberry Balsamic
        Dressing, 84, *85*
    Ranch Dressing, 7, 79, 183
    salad bar, 78
    Sesame Red Cabbage & Carrot Slaw, 76, *77*
    Super Salad with Garlic Caesar Dressing & Hemp
        Hearts, *82*, 83

Salsa, *40*, 41
Salt, 7
Sample menus, 220–3
Sandwiches, burgers and wraps, 86–7
    Beans & Greens Quesadillas, *100*, 101
    Beetroot Burgers, 98, *99*
    Black Bean Burgers, 88, *89*
    Curried Chickpea Wraps, 92, *93*
    Sloppy Jacks, *90*, 91
    Spinach & Mushroom Black Bean Burritos, 94, *95*
    Veracruz Tempeh Lettuce Wraps, *96*, 97
Sauces
    Almond Butter Sauce, 146
    Arrabiata, 108, *109*
    Avocado-Cashew Alfredo, *104*, 105
    Balsamic-Date Glaze, 8, 176, *177*
    Berry Drizzle, 16, *17*
    Black Bean Sauce, *154*, 155
    Blackberry Coulis, 192, *193*
    Chermoula Sauce, 118, *119*
    Golden Gravy, 156–7, *157*
    Harissa, 9, 138, *139*
    Herbed Mushroom Gravy, 112, *113*
    Lemon Tahini Sauce, *114*, 115
    Lentil Bolognese, 150, *151*
    Spicy Ginger Sauce, 128, *129*
    Tomato-Red Pepper Coulis, 116, *117*
    Umami Sauce, xxii, 5, 27
    Warm Pear Compote, 18, *19*
    Yellow Pepper Béarnaise, 164, *165*
Savory Spice Blend, xxii, 4, 6, 7, 9, 24, 27, 30, 35, 36, 38,
    41, 44, 48, 51, 52, 54, 56, 59, 60, 63, 64, 66, 70,
    72, 83, 88, 91, 92, 94, 101, 108, 115, 127, 137,
    143, 149, 167, 180, 183
Seaweed, 51
Seeds. *See* Nuts and seeds
Sesame Red Cabbage & Carrot Slaw, 76, 77
Shopping, 227–9
Side dishes, 162–3
    Baked Onion Rings, 180, *181*
    Buffalo Cauliflower, 7, 183
    Cauliflower Mash, *174*, 175
    Garlic Greens Sauté, 178
    Indian-Style Spinach and Tomatoes, 170, *171*

    Lemon-Roasted Brussels Sprouts & Carrots with
        Pecans, *166*, 167
    Red Cabbage Sauté, *172*, 173
    Roasted Asparagus with Yellow Pepper Béarnaise,
        164, *165*
    Roasted Beetroots with Balsamic-Braised Beetroot
        Greens, 168
    Stuffed Sweet Potatoes, 8, 176, *177*
Silicone mats, 225
Simmering, 225
60 Minutes, xi
Sloppy Jacks, *90*, 91
Smoked meat, xvii
Smoked paprika, 63
Smoky Roasted Chickpeas, 44, *45*
Smoothies
    Banana-Chocolate Smoothie, 210, *211*
    Cherry-Berry Smoothie, *214*, 215
    Pumpkin Pie Smoothie, 212, *213*
    Super Green Smoothie, 216, *217*
    V-12 Vegetable Blast, *218*, 219
Snacks, 28–9
    Artichoke-Spinach Dip, 30, *31*
    Black-Eyed Peas & Roasted Red Pepper Dip, 36, *37*
    Cheesy Kale Crisps, 42, *43*
    Edamame Guacamole, 38, *39*
    fruit, as, 41
    Lemony Hummus, *32*, 33
    popcorn, 44
    Pumpkin Seed Dip, 35
    Smoky Roasted Chickpeas, 44, *45*
    Summer Salsa, 40, 41
    Three-Seed Crackers, 34
Soda, xvi
Sodium, 7
Soups and chillies, 46–7
    Black Bean Soup with Quinoa & Kale, 56, *57*
    Champion Vegetable Chilli, 66, *67*
    Curried Cauliflower Soup, 58, *59*
    Kale & White Bean Soup, 48, *49*
    Miso Soup with Spinach & Dulse, 51
    Moroccan Lentil Soup, 63
    Spicy Asian Vegetable Soup, 52, *53*
    Summer Garden Gazpacho, 60, *61*

Three-Bean Chilli, 64, *65*
Vegetable Broth, 6
Vegetable & Red Bean Gumbo, 54, *55*
Soyabean foods, 98
    Braised Tempeh & Bok Choy with Spicy Ginger
        Sauce, 128, *129*
    Buckwheat Soba & Edamame with Almond Butter
        Sauce, 146
    Edamame Guacamole, 38, *39*
    Louisiana Soy Curls, *136*, 137
    miso, 7, 51
    steaming tempeh, 225
    Veracruz Tempeh Lettuce Wraps, *96*, 97
Spaghetti Squash Arrabiata, 108, *109*
Spices. *See also* Curry powder; Turmeric
    cardamom, 63
    cinnamon, 63
    cooking tips for, 2
    cooking with, 63
    paprika, 63
    saffron, xviii
    Savory Spice Blend, xxii, 4, 27
Spicy Asian Vegetable Soup, 52, *53*
Spicy Ginger Sauce, 128, *129*
Spinach
    Artichoke-Spinach Dip, 30, *31*
    as cancer-fighting food, 95
    for diseases, 95
    Indian-Style Spinach and Tomatoes, 170, *171*
    Miso Soup with Spinach & Dulse, 51
    Pistachio-Spinach Salad with Strawberry Balsamic
        Dressing, 84, *85*
    Spinach & Mushroom Black Bean Burritos, 94, *95*
    using, 94
Spreads. *See* Dips and spreads
Spring Greens
    Hoppin' John Stuffed Spring Greens Rolls, 158, *159*
    Smoky Black-Eyed Peas & Spring Greens, *126*, 127
Squash
    Courgette Noodles with Avocado-Cashew Alfredo,
        104, 105
    Pumpkin Pie Smoothie, 212, *213*
    Spaghetti Squash Arrabiata, 108, *109*
Stuffed Winter Squash with Black Bean Sauce, 154, *155*
Steaming, 225

Stir-frying, 226
Stomach cancer, 7
Storage containers, 33
Strawberries
    Strawberry Balsamic Dressing, 84, *85*
    Strawberry-Banana Nice Cream, *196*, 197
Stroke, xiii–xiv, xvi
Stuffed Portobellos with Herbed Mushroom Gravy, 112,
    113
Stuffed Sweet Potatoes, 8, 176, *177*
Sugar, date, 3
Suicidal depression, xviii
Summer Garden Gazpacho, 60, *61*
Summer Salsa, 40, 41
Summertime Oatmeal, 12, *13*
Super Green Smoothie, 216, *217*
Super Salad with Garlic Caesar Dressing & Hemp
    Hearts, *82*, 83
Superfood Breakfast Bites, 14, 15
Sweet Potatoes
    Burrito Breakfast Bake, 24, *25*
    Frying Pan Sweet Potato Hash, *26*, 27
    Stuffed Sweet Potatoes, 8, 176, *177*
Sweets. *See* Desserts and sweets
Syrup, 3, 22, *23*

T

Tabbouleh, 70, *71*
Tagine, 124, *125*
Tahini, *114*, 115
Teff, 98
Tempeh
    Braised Tempeh & Bok Choy with Spicy Ginger
        Sauce, 128, *129*
    steaming, 225
    Veracruz Tempeh Lettuce Wraps, *96*, 97
Tetra Pak, 24
Three-Bean Chilli, 64, *65*
Three-Seed Crackers, 34
Time-saving cooking tips, 2
Tomato products, 229
Tomatoes

Indian-Style Spinach and Tomatoes, 170, *171*
Pesto Carrot Noodles with White Beans & Tomatoes, 106, *107*
Summer Garden Gazpacho, 60, *61*
Summer Salsa, *40*, 41
Tomato-Red Pepper Coulis, 116, *117*
Tortillas, 229
Toxic heavy metals, xix
Traffic-light classification system, x–xi, 2
Triglyceride levels, 8
Turmeric
    as cancer-fighting food, xiv
    for diseases, 70
    in French Toast with Berry Drizzle, 16
    in Golden Gravy, 156–7, *157*
    in Golden Quinoa Tabbouleh, 70, *71*
    ten ways to eat, 70
Two-Berry Pie with Pecan-Sunflower Crust, *202*, 203
Type 2 diabetes
    diet and, viii–ix
    insulin in, xv
    kidney disease and, xv
    medications for, viii–x, xvi
    type 2, viii–ix
    whole-food, plant-based nutrition for, xv–xvi

Umami, 5
Umami Sauce, xxii, 5, 27, 64, 121, 128, 133, 144, 146, 155, 173,

V

V-12 Vegetable Blast, *218*, 219
Veganism, x
Vegetable Broth, 5, 6, 30, 48, 51, 52, 54, 56, 59, 63, 64, 66, 105, 106, 112, 124, 128, 130, 133, 134, 137, 143, 152, 155, 157, 164, 173, 178, 226
Vegetable & Red Bean Gumbo, 54, *55*

Vegetable Stacks with Tomato-Red Pepper Coulis, 116, *117*
Vegetable Unfried Rice, 144, *145*
Vegetarianism, x
Veracruz Tempeh Lettuce Wraps, *96*, 97
Vinegar, 5, 73
    Balsamic-Braised Beetroot Greens, 168
    Balsamic-Date Glaze, 8, 176, *177*
    Strawberry Balsamic Dressing, 84, *85*
Vision loss, xv

Walnuts, 106
    No-Bake Oatmeal Walnut Cookies, *188*, 189
Warm Pear Compote, 18, *19*
Water, 206
Watercress, 134, *135*
Water-sauté, 226
Weight, xv, 92
Wheat. *See* Grains
White beans
    Kale & White Bean Soup, 48, *49*
    Pesto Carrot Noodles with White Beans & Tomatoes, 106, *107*
White blood cells, xv
White rice, x
Whole Roasted Cauliflower with Lemon Tahini Sauce, *114*, 115
Whole-food, plant-based nutrition, x–xi
    for blood cancers, xvii
    for brain diseases, xiii–xiv
    for breast cancer, xvii–xviii
    for coronary heart disease, xi, xii–xiii
    for digestive cancers, xiv–xv
    diseases and, xi
    for high blood pressure, xvi
    for infections, xv
    for kidney disease, xvii
    for liver disease, xvi
    for lung diseases, xiii
    for Parkinson's disease, xix

for prostate cancer, xviii
for suicidal depression, xviii
for type 2 diabetes, xv–xvi
weight and, xv
Womb, xiii
Wraps
Beans & Greens Quesadillas, *100*, 101
Curried Chickpea Wraps, 92, *93*
Spinach & Mushroom Black Bean Burritos, 94, *95*
Veracruz Tempeh Lettuce Wraps, *96*, 97

Y

Yeast, nutritional, 4, 44
Yellow Light foods, xi, 2
Yellow Pepper Béarnaise, 164, *165*
Yellow Rice & Black Beans with Broccoli, 152, *153*